The Complete Gastric Sleeve Bariatric Cookbook

Easy Guidance with Meal Plan & Healthy Recipes to Eat Well & Keep the Weight Off after Weight-Loss Surgery

By Nigel Methews

ISBN: 9798736811915

Table of Contents

INTRODUCTION

For some individuals, at times, optimizing weight loss is just not possible, no matter how hard they try. So, it becomes important to try some permanent fix for their dietary habits. Dietary restrictions recommended for weight loss do not work for everyone, as some people can stick to the same routine throughout their lives. Now there are permanent weight loss solutions that can make life easy for those who have genetic tendencies to gain weight quickly or have a naturally slow metabolism. Bariatric treatment includes methods that can reduce the size of the stomach in order to restrict food consumption. Gastric Sleeve Surgery is among those methods, which is considered most effective with lesser complications and health risks. If you are planning on getting this surgery and want some great information to prepare your mind for the process, then this book can help you big time! And you have already gone through the process; the dietary guidelines will help you create a new menu and will help you learn all the lifestyle changes that are required to live a healthy life after Gastric Sleeve Surgery. In this gastric sleeve diet cookbook, you will learn all about the gastric sleeve diet and the relevant recipes that you can add to your new lifestyle.

CHAPTER 1: Welcome to the Sleeve Club

If you are reading this book, you must have gone through the vertical sleeve gastrectomy (VSG) or are planning to get it soon. I know the thought of having surgery sparks so many doubts and confusion in our minds. The idea of permanently reducing the size of your stomach is too big to comprehend. It is therefore important to fully understand this concept and learn what you should be expecting after the surgery. With the right combination of food, prescribed dietary changes, and an active lifestyle, you can have successful results after this treatment. What you need is smart planning and a will to make this happen. Ask yourself, *Am I ready for this?* If there are some concerns that you have about this surgery and your life after it, then continue to read on, as I am about to share a detailed account of the VSG and the diet that you need to follow after this treatment.

What is the Vertical Sleeve Gastrectomy?

Vertical sleeve gastrectomy, or sleeve surgery, is a process in which the stomach's capacity to hold the food is reduced by 80 percent. In other words, a sleeve is created on the side of the stomach, which receives the food in a small amount; the rest is separated through this surgery. This bariatric procedure is also called weight-loss surgery, as it is used to induce weight loss through a permanent approach. This surgical method to reduce the stomach size only works when the post-surgery lifestyle is supported by a healthy diet and active routine. For this reason, a complete progressive diet plan is suggested for people who go through this surgery. The bariatric treatments are not new to medical sciences; the concept had been under debate and discussion for quite some time. But it was not until January 1, 2010, that United Healthcare added the gastric sleeve surgery to their list of surgeries that they started to provide for weight loss. And, approximately two years later, all other renowned health insurance companies started to cover the bariatric procedure. It is not easy to make health insurance companies approve new surgical treatments since there are several risks involved, but gastric sleeve surgery was readily approved because the evidence suggested that the procedure could result in significant results in terms of weight loss. And it was also confirmed that the surgery has minimum complications and risks compared to other bariatric surgeries.

Why Get Sleeved?

The gastric sleeve surgery is mainly opted for to achieve weight loss. This surgery works for people who are sensitive to dietary changes and just can't lose weight through diet control. So, this surgery finds a permanent solution and reduces the stomach size, which automatically cuts down food consumption.

This surgery has given effective results, and within one year of the surgery, people should experience 70 percent weight loss. By controlling obesity, such individuals were also able to resist diabetes, insulin resistance, sleep apnea, hypertension, joint pain, fatty liver disease, and hyperlipidemia. Excessive hunger sensations are also reduced to a minimum after gastric sleeve surgery. The procedure is indeed effective, but it works well only when a person changes his dietary habits after the surgery and follows a gastric sleeve diet.

In this stomach reduction treatment, the surgeon removes a wide portion of the stomach and turns it into a narrow tube or "sleeve" connecting the two ends. The new, narrow banana-shaped stomach turns out to be smaller than the original size of the stomach. The removed part of the stomach that is separated basically promotes the production of hormones that help increase appetite and control the production of insulin. So, after the sleeve surgery, a person's appetite potentially decreases, and any signs of insulin resistance are reduced. The person then eats less, feels full after eating a small amount, and does not get frequent hunger pangs. This process is quite effective, but it is not reversible.

This surgery is carried out to help people achieve weight loss and to prevent weight gain. This procedure is recommended to people who are severely overweight and, despite all efforts, haven't been able to lose weight, either through exercise, diet, or medicine. And most of the time, those people are not even binge eating or emotional eating. Sometimes it is really not just in your hands or in your conscious control. Everyone's body works differently, and no one can judge others through his or her eating practices.

Even though the stomach after the surgery can again stretch out to accommodate food, this operation makes the patient feel less hungry, and they consume less food so their weight is controlled. People willing to opt for this procedure should have a body mass index ranging between 40–60 and higher. They should be having weight-caused health or life-damaging problems. Studies indicate that obese people who go through this surgery are at lesser risk of developing cancer, diabetes, and heart problems than those obese people who do not lose weight.

The sleeve gastrectomy is considered less risky than a gastric bypass because, in this procedure, the small intestine is not divided or reconnected to create a bypass in order to decrease its size. The main risks and complications that could need another operation stand to be 5 percent. Today, gastric sleeve surgery is used as the only gastric procedure to perform on patients; it is still often used as part of a great gastric treatment and approach to deal with weight loss. In such approaches, the surgery is followed by an intestinal rerouting or a bypass operation. However, the weight loss that is gained as a result of the sleeve gastrectomy surgery makes this intestinal bypass unnecessary.

Often, a surgeon who plans to perform a gastric bypass procedure initially has a change of mind and instead opts for the gastric sleeve procedure, as the bypass procedure can cause liver enlargement or extensive scars on the tissues of the intestines, which makes the gastric bypass almost impossible, among other reasons people usually get the sleeve gastrectomy to include Crohn's disease, severe body comorbidities, aging, continuous medications, monitoring of the stomach and its functionality, or all the risks combined together to cause more complications.

Starting Over Food

What a patient does after the surgery makes all the difference. If he continues to eat like before and lives a sedentary lifestyle, then even this surgery isn't going to help him much. Following are some important tips that must be kept in mind to lead a healthy and active life after the surgery.

1. Keep the portion sizes in check

It is healthy to eat meals slowly and to measure the quantity of food that you are consuming. Eating too fast might lead to overeating, and this will take you to the failure of your weight loss goals.

2. Have more protein in your diet

Consumption of a good amount of protein daily after the gastric sleeve surgery will help the patient heal faster; it also helps to prevent the possible loss of muscle mass and also helps to maintain the body's energy levels. The carbohydrate meal is digested faster and reduces hunger, but when instead of carbohydrates, protein is broken down slowly, the patient keeps feeling full.

3. Rely on vitamins and nutritional supplements

After this sleeve surgery, you may need to reduce meal intake to four ounces. This means that you need to meet your nutritional needs with supplement vitamins and minerals. You can also experience difficulty in absorbing vitamin B1, B6, and B12, so vitamin supplementation is necessary after this gastric surgery.

4. Be physically active

Regular routine exercise is one of the ways that can help you to maintain your body weight for the long term. It also helps to alleviate the risks of chronic diseases like cancer, diabetes, and heart disease. It also helps to improve the body's flexibility.

5. Stay hydrated all the time

To keep your body functions normal, like body temperature, kidney functions, blood pressure, and healthy skin, you need to always keep the body hydrated. Drink plenty of water during the day, as it will help you to keep hydrated and also control appetite by keeping the stomach full.

6. Eating habits and lifestyle changes

The long-term success of weight-loss surgery entirely depends on your willingness to change your routine habits. These habits include increasing physical activities, controlling daily food intake, focusing on the intake of protein, etc. Start by adopting new eating habits that can help you to keep the weight off.

7. Avoid high caloric drinks

Avoid all beverages high in calories and drink only low-calorie drinks like sugar-free juices, water, and unsweetened iced tea. Some people do not lose their weight even after four months of the surgery only because they keep consuming sugar and carbs through their drinks.

Food Texture Week by week

After having the surgery, you will need to gradually switch to solid food. For this reason, each week, the diet calls for a change in food texture and variety. Here is how the food form and variety change every week for your bariatric post-op diet:

The Clear Liquids

This stage begins in the first week after the gastric sleeve surgery. Since the stomach is newly stapled or stitch, it cannot bear any solid food in it. Therefore, liquids that can run down the digestive tract without needing any digestion are needed. In this stage of the diet, only a few ounces of liquid food are allowed. This will help your stomach heal without becoming stretched by foods. The liquid diet includes:

1. Water
2. Soup and broth
3. Skim milk
4. Decaffeinated coffee and tea
5. Sugar-free gelatin and popsicles
6. Unsweetened juice

Avoid all the sugary drinks and liquids during this first stage after gastric sleeve surgery. Consuming sugary drinks may lead to an increase in digestive problems and can lead to negative side effects from sleeve surgery. The patient must also avoid carbonated and caffeinated beverages. During this stage, after the surgery, it is advised to keep the body hydrated; therefore, it is important to constantly drink a small amount of liquid at a time.

Protein-Rich Liquids

Now that the stomach has started to heal, the patient can move to liquids, which also contain nutrients. This second stage begins five to seven days after the gastric sleeve surgery. The time of healing varies for individuals; therefore, one week is set as a standard criterion to move to the second stage. During this stage, you have to consume protein-rich shakes and liquids that included skimmed milk, unsweetened, and blended fruit juice. During this stage, you will experience a minute increase in your appetite, but you have to stick to your diet plan to get a positive result. The protein-rich liquid includes:

1. Sugar-free protein shakes
2. Low-carb yogurt
3. Thin creamed soup and broth
4. Split pea or lentil soup
5. All food in stage one

During the second stage, it is recommended to consume nearly three liters of liquids per day. Avoid consuming sugary and carbonated liquids during this stage.

Pureed Diet

The next stage takes you from liquids to pureed solids. Stage three begins nearly after two weeks of gastric sleeve surgery. It allows the patient to include pureed soft food into the diet. The foods may include mashed potatoes, fat-free yogurts, thick and smooth soups, baked beans, etc. You are allowed to eat these light food items in small quantities about five times daily. Food that is allowed at this stage includes:

1. Tofu
2. Pureed sugar-free fruits
3. Pureed peas and lentils
4. Eggs
5. Plain yogurt
6. Steamed or boiled vegetables

Remember that whatever food you are consuming must be pureed after the required cooking.

Solid Food

The final stage is the actual stage that will lead you to a healthy diet that will progress throughout your post gastric sleeve surgery diet. It begins after the four weeks of gastric sleeve surgery. It allows you to consume soft solid food in the diet. Try to consume high-protein foods because it recommends having at least 60 grams of protein in daily meals. During this stage, the stomach is healed enough and should handle solid food. During this fourth stage, you can have three meals in a day with some light and healthy snacks in between the meals. The solid foods that are allowed in this stage include:

1. Fish
2. Lentil and beans soup
3. Hot cereals
4. Boiled potatoes
5. Cooked vegetables

6. Low-fat cheese

7. Lean ground turkey, chicken, beef, pork

8. Soft fruits without skin

At this stage, you must avoid oily snacks; whole milk products; sugary drinks; extremely fibrous vegetables like broccoli, celery, and asparagus; starchy foods like white potatoes; spicy foods; pasta; bread; processed and fried fast-food, etc.

VSG Nutritional Know-How

Malnutrition is possible in both gastric sleeve and gastric bypass patients, especially if supplements are not taken. Deficiencies for which you will need to compensate for with supplements for the rest of your life following your gastric surgery include the following. You should look for food that is rich in these nutrients so that you will not suffer from their deficiencies.

Calcium and Vitamin D

A decrease in calcium, vitamin D, and exercise will eventually result in bone resorption and osteoporosis.

Iron

Iron is the vital element for red blood cell production, for liver parenchymal cells, and for the reticuloendothelial system. Iron deficiency anemia will occur if supplements are not taken, especially in women of reproductive age who are menstruating.

Vitamin B12

Deficiency in vitamin B12 results in emotional changes like depression, psychosis, depression, decreased cognitive capabilities, poor motor function, changes in nervous reflexes, low red blood cells, decreased fertility, reduced heart function, inflammation of the tongue, and decreased taste. Folate is a B vitamin; it makes and repairs DNA and produces red blood cells. A deficiency of this vitamin results in anemia, which deprives your tissues of oxygen and then affects their function. Birth defects are sometimes caused by folate deficiency during pregnancy. Folate deficiency symptoms include growth problems, tongue swelling, mouth sores, gray hair, and fatigue. Folate deficiency leads to anemia, which has symptoms of irritability, shortness of breath, pale skin, lethargy, weakness, and persistent fatigue. Fortified cereals, fruits, and vegetables contain folate.

Vitamin A

Night blindness is caused by a lack of vitamin A in the diet, as is a diminished ability to fight off infections and maternal mortality.

Selenium

Insufficient selenium results in muscle wasting, muscle myopathy, arrhythmia, cardiomyopathy, reduced thyroid, and immunity function. Loss of hair and skin pigment can also occur, along with encephalopathy and white nail beds. Absorption of selenium is helped along with vitamins C and E.

Vitamin E

Deficiency in vitamin E causes neurological and neuromuscular problems, anemia, retinopathy, and impairment of the immune response.

Vitamin K

A lack of vitamin K can result in massive uncontrolled bleeding, bleeding at the surgical sites, stomach pains, cartilage calcification, and malformation of developing bone. This vitamin is used by the liver to create enzymes needed for the coagulation of the blood.

Protein

Protein prevents hair loss, sickness, flaky dermatitis, and fluid retention in the ankles and feet. Protein keeps bones, skin, nails, and hair healthy. Malabsorption can also lead to kidney oxalate stones and lactic acidosis. Most importantly, for the gastric sleeve patient, protein aids in proper wound healing and promotes weight loss. Protein helps with weight loss in several ways. It satisfies and therefore discourages a dieter from eating extra calories due to hunger. Protein helps a person to feel full, strong, and energized because protein takes longer to digest than carbs and some other foods do.

Know how important proteins are for this diet. Proteins were named after the Greek word proteins, which literally means prime importance. It is undoubtedly the most important nutrient in the gastric bariatric diet. Protein is a part of each cell of the body, and these proteins are continuously broken down, repaired, and reproduced by the cells. Since the body cannot store protein for longer use, constantly consuming high-quality protein is the basic need of every individual, especially those who are recovering from gastric sleeve surgery. When protein intake is not sufficient, the body breaks down body mass to offset the body's muscle mass.

As the loss of lean body mass is always inevitable, especially after gastric sleeve surgery due to minimized calorie intake, you can prevent this by taking in a high amount of good-quality protein daily. Protein can help in the healing of the wound after bariatric surgery. It helps to build and repair all the body tissues, which include skin and muscle repair. Protein also helps the body to burn fat instead of muscle for a healthier weight loss.

As you step into Stage 4 of this diet and beyond, you will start incorporating more solid proteins into your daily diet. Look out for food sources, which will keep you feeling fuller for a longer duration of time. Liquid or soft food should only be used as a protein source until the third week after the surgery; this may include all protein-rich shakes, dairy yogurt, or cottage cheese.

However, the solid sources of protein contain all the eggs, meat, and some lentils. About four-and-a-half ounces of chicken with a protein shake together can provide 30 grams of protein, which is an optimal intake for the fourth stage and beyond. The chicken and poultry will make you feel full for a longer duration of time than the protein shake.

Intake of Incomplete and Complete Proteins

Proteins are made up of amino acids that are used for every metabolic process in the body, whether anabolic or catabolic. Amino acids are basically the building units of protein and of the body too. For good health, there are nine essential amino acids that are not produced in the body, so a person may need to receive those from dietary sources. Due to the difference between amino acids, not all proteins are the same. The bariatric diet patient should have a primary goal to get high-quality protein food to meet all the nutritional needs. Many patients may get confused as to which types of protein they should consume and what is considered a good protein food. The theory of complete and incomplete proteins can help understand the difference.

Sources that provide nothing but all the essential amino acids in their proteins are known as complete protein sources. All animal-based proteins are termed complete proteins because they are full of all nine of the essential amino acids required by the body, which mainly include the following options:

1. Seafood and Fish
2. Beef

3. Poultry

4. Pork

5. Eggs

6. Dairy

Sources that cannot provide all nine essential amino acids in a single protein are known as incomplete proteins. All plant-based proteins are termed incomplete proteins because they lack at least one or more of the nine amino acids that our body needs the most. The following are incomplete protein options:

1. Beans, including pinto, kidney, garbanzo, chickpeas, etc.

2. All lentils and split pea

3. All nuts and seeds

4. All forms of grains and rice

5. All vegetables

Increase your Protein Intake

The calories from protein sources vary from source to source; it all depends on the fat and carbohydrate content that is present in the food besides the proteins. When you are choosing protein, look for sources high in protein grams and low in calories to maximize nutrition and keep calories low for weight loss and maintenance. Use a guideline to make your decision, and consume a minimum of 10 grams of protein for every 100 calories. The higher the protein intake and the lower the calories in the food, the better the diet will be. This formula is one good way to assess the quality of the protein-based diet and to determine if it is suitable for your health or not.

To maximize your daily protein intake and to make it 60 grams per day, you can use the following ingredients as a major source of all the complete proteins and essential amino acids:

1. Cottage cheese
2. Protein shake
3. Chicken
4. Halibut
5. String cheese
6. Ribeye
7. Chicken sausage
8. Mozzarella cheese
9. Almonds
10. Peanut butter
11. Black beans
12. Cheddar cheese

The 10 percent limit can be taken as a guideline to maximize daily protein intake. For every 100 calories you consume, a minimum of 10 grams should be consumed from lean, good-quality protein sources. Make sure it is 60 grams per day. This limit is set to keep your meals focused and to maintain protein intake each day while keeping your calories low to achieve your weight loss goals. Weight loss may be slowed down or will eventually stop if the daily caloric intake reaches 1,000 or more per day.

The Bariatric Kitchen

Your life after this surgery is going to change altogether. You will have to set up your pantry according to the new lifestyle and the diet that can best support your gut and digestive system. There are certain things that you must have in your bariatric kitchen. The items are categorized into pre- and post-surgery lists, and you should arrange them accordingly to stay prepared. Besides food, you will also need to keep some supplements in your kitchen to have complete nutrients on this diet.

Pre-Surgery Grocery List

1. Beans
2. Applesauce
3. Canned meat or fish in water
4. Broth
5. Canned fruit packed in water
6. Cream of wheat cereal
7. Cream soup
8. Cottage cheese
9. Eggs
10. Hummus
11. Milk (skim, 1%)
12. Jell-O (sugar-free)
13. Oatmeal (plain)
14. Oat bran cereal
15. Pudding (low fat, no sugar added)
16. Lentils (canned)
17. Soda crackers or melba toast
18. Soy milk (unsweetened)
19. Yogurt, Greek or regular

20. Skim milk powder

21. Zero-calorie drinks

Post-Surgery Grocery List

1. Bone broth

2. Herbal teas

3. Matcha maker green tea

4. Coconut water

5. Springwater

6. Sugar-free Jell-O gelatin

7. Sugar-free popsicles

8. Green juice diluted with water

9. Juice diluted with springwater

10. Almond milk

11. Strained soups

Supplements for VSG

1. Flintstones Complete

2. One-A-Day Maximum

3. Solara Calcium Citrate Wafers

4. Chewable Mega Teen Multivitamin

5. Citrucel Creamy Bites

6. Twin Labs Chewable Calcium Citrate

7. Centrum Chewable

8. Calcium with Vitamin D

9. Bluebonnet Liquid Calcium Citrate

10. Protein-rich foods

Foods to Avoid after Surgery

Sugar and carbs can easily ruin all your weight loss efforts, and so do the bad fats (or sometimes even the good fats) if eaten in excess. On the gastric sleeve diet, it is recommended to avoid that food that the stomach and intestines are not capable of digesting in a short time. Avoid the following foods to prevent sabotaging your weight loss efforts:

1. Doughnuts

2. Fried food

3. Alcohol

4. Ice cream

5. Preserves

6. Flavoured drink mix

7. Sherbet

8. Cakes

9. Molasses

10. Honey

11. Regular sodas

12. Sweets

13. Candy

CHAPTER 2: VSG Meal Plans

Meal plans are as important as the surgery itself because once you get through this, only a feasible and practical meal plan will help you achieve the true benefits of this surgery and the diet. As you can feel full quickly eating after this surgery, you should eat between two and four ounces of food and drink up to six times a day; it is a good amount to start out with. Then, gradually work up to consume a little more food over time. Add non-fat dry milk powder whenever you can. Your protein goal is 70 grams per day. Meal planning can help you big time if you are on a gastric sleeve diet. It has the following benefits to look for:

Time-Saver

When you don't get enough time in a day to work and enjoy a good meal, it is ideal to meal prep beforehand to save your time and health too. Meal prep is quite time-effective; by spending one or two days in the kitchen, you can prepare food for an entire week. This also saves you from the worries of constantly deciding on the right dish at the right time.

Budget-Friendly

Those of you who work every day end up hitting the nearest restaurant, a food chain, or a store to buy ready-made products. These items are costly when you compare the quality of home-cooked food. Meal prepping saves you from such wastage of money and gives you better alternatives. Moreover, by listing ingredients as per each day, you only buy what you eat, not what you would eat or things that are later discarded because they're spoiled.

Health Effective

Homemade food is the healthiest of all. You select the ingredients as per the quality and then bring them together to cook a nice luscious meal. Meal prepping saves us from ordering junk to eat and leaves us with a home-cooked meal, which is healthy to the core. This is why meal prepping is known for the good nutritional values it provides to every individual.

Controlled Metabolism

Our metabolism does not remain the same throughout the day; it varies from person to person and from time to time. With meal prepping, you can eat, taking your metabolism into consideration. If you are bogged down with physical work, you can add high-energy food to the menu, whereas for lazy days, you can reduce the amount of fat and carb intake to meet your needs accordingly; in this way, it maintains our metabolism.

Meal Planning Errors to Avoid

Initially, we cannot become a pro at anything; with time and practice, we adopt certain habits. Meal prepping is a gradual process that also takes experience. Making mistakes, in the beginning, is quite natural; however, with certain tips and care, you can avoid a few of the basic errors that every beginner commits. These are:

Poor or No Labeling

Once food is stored and frozen, it's hard to differentiate between some, as they look quite similar. Plus, there can be a mix-up between breakfast, lunch, and dinner. So, avoid it all, and try labeling the container with their names and the days.

Using Fewer Ingredients

Often, beginners buy groceries randomly and then make up their minds about meal prepping. In the end, they find most of the items not suitable for good use. Or they don't have items that would be essential for meal prepping. This is why mental work is most important. First, write down the complete list of ingredients that you will need for the rest of the week, and then go to the store.

Over-Preparation

"Excess of everything is not good." This adage also fits in this scenario because sometimes people cook an extra meal, which can get wasted. Cook only for a week; otherwise, the stored food will not turn out to be as healthy and nutritious as it originally was. Prepare only what you can eat and store as much needed, not more than that.

Inappropriate Containers

Storing food is important, and for that, it is essential to use the right type of container. Use as many containers as are required. Store every meal in a different box. Seal them properly. Keep a container of different sizes to store food as per the size of the servings. You can also use Ziplock bags to store food if needed.

No Refrigeration

One storage capacity that matters the most is freezer storage. Without sufficient space in the freezer, storing can't be effective. People often overstuff their freezers, which affects the cooling of the refrigerator. Avoid this by first creating sufficient space, then placing the container inside.

Planning for an Extended Time Period

If you are not willing to give sufficient time to the meal preparation, it won't be as delicious and healthy as you expect it. Preparing a meal for a whole week is not a one-hour job; it takes at least a few hours and an interruption in your normal routine. All these efforts are totally worth it.

Weekly Meal Plan for VSG

The following is how you can successfully execute a bariatric diet meal according to your improving condition and the changing form of food required to support your surgical changes and new lifestyle.

First Day

A radiologist soon gives the patient a swallow test that will look for the major leaks in the stomach area before he will be allowed by the surgeon to have water to drink. He should only have a small amount of anything on this day. No carbonated drinks or drinks with caffeine will be allowed on this day. Caffeine creates a diuretic effect, which is a major reason that patients who cheat and drink something with caffeine are readmitted because of dehydration!

Don't accept drinks or food from well-meaning family or friends that are not on the list of allowed drinks or food. Follow the doctor's orders. There is a good reason for not consuming whatever he tells you not to consume! You will likely just be thirsty on this day, but if you do want something other than water, your choices will be as follows:

1. Sugar-free gelatin
2. Strained cream soup
3. Milk
4. Unsweetened juice
5. Broth

Initial Days after the Surgery

You will need to get whatever you consume on your own unless you have children or unemployed friends lined up to help you after you get home. What you are allowed to eat during these two days is up to your surgeon. You may still be on the liquid diet for the remainder of the week. Alternatively, you may be allowed to advance to pureed food at some point during your first week following surgery. If you can have pureed food, it cannot have lumps in it. The food allowed will likely include the following items:

1. Yogurt
2. Lean ground meat
3. Fish
4. Soft fruit
5. Beans
   Liquids allowed on this diet mainly include the following:
6. Juice
7. Fat-free milk
8. Broth
9. Water

Your body is used to receive a lot of its fluids from food, but it won't get all that it needs from food now. You need to drink a lot of fluids from now on. Check your sugar levels if you are diabetic. Your diabetes meds have likely been reduced now as part of the discharge plan.

First-Week Plan

As previously discussed, you won't have much desire to eat food right after the surgery because the hunger hormone ghrelin is not produced in you. That is because the area of the stomach where most of that hormone was produced has now been removed. Stay on the clear liquid diet by days two and three. You cannot have caffeine, sugar, or sweet beverages. You may not have carbonated beverages at this stage, so the clear-liquid options that you can consume during this early time period consist of the following:

1. Decaffeinated coffee
2. Sugar-free drinks
3. Sugar-free popsicles
4. Decaffeinated tea
5. Jell-O
6. Broth
7. Water

Second-Week Plan

You may actually start feeling a little hungry by now, but it will be a week that will make you want more of the tasty protein shakes. Hopefully, you pre-made, tested, tweaked, and froze a bunch of different flavors of shakes and smoothies before your surgery. Hopefully, the family has stayed out of them too! Eat whatever the surgeon tells you to eat, but your diet will likely include the following choices:

1. Protein powder mixed with a clear liquid that is sugar-free and noncarbonated
2. Non-fat yogurt
3. Cream soups thinned out with water and containing no chunks in it

4. Sugar-free sorbet

5. Soups with soft noodles

6. Diluted, no-sugar-added juice

7. Sugar-free pudding

8. Sugar-free and very watery hot oatmeal

9. Thinned applesauce with no sugar added

Third-Week Plan

This week will get a bit tough for you. You will be able to add some normal food to your diet; though pureed, some of it can make you sick. Some food may taste different to you now. Some food may not be tolerated well after your surgery, such as dairy. If you introduce the food gradually, you will be able to find food that you have trouble with so as to avoid it for a while.

You must also need to write what types of food are making you feel sick. Did it cause or upset your stomach, or has it caused diarrhea? If it is your homemade shakes, determine what you can put into the shakes so that you can document the ingredients from which one or more may not yet agree with your new digestive system. Continue to limit sugar and fat. This week you have three goals you need to reach, which are:

Consume about 60 grams of protein each day; increase this amount if you are a man. Eat your food slowly. Introduce new food one at a time, but not during the same meal. During this week, you need to avoid the following items: Fibrous vegetables such as broccoli, celery, asparagus, and raw leafy greens. Also, avoid starchy foods like pasta, rice, and bread.

Even your protein smoothies and shakes can have too much sugar in the form of fructose, so you may need to consume those extra-fruity drinks in smaller doses than the other smoothies and shakes during this stage.

Food choices for this week include the following items:

1. Hummus

2. Coconut milk in shakes

3. Low-fat cottage cheese

4. One smoothie

5. Soft cereal

6. Soft cheeses in a limited amount

7. Soft steamed or boiled vegetables

8. Ground beef mixed with stock to keep it soft

9. Ground chicken mixed with stock to keep it soft

10. Soups

11. Scrambled eggs, use them as a good source of protein

12. Canned tuna mixed with low-fat mayonnaise, again a good source of protein

13. Canned salmon mixed with low-fat mayonnaise, an extremely good source of protein

14. Mashed fruit that has not had sugar added to it (bananas are great)

15. Mashed avocados

Week Four: Eat Real Food

Well, you do not have to eat pureed food this week! You still need to eat softer versions of the various food options, and you need to continue to chew your food well. Your stomach is still sensitive. You need to avoid the following food items:

1. Sodas
2. Fried foods
3. Sugary drinks
4. Candy
5. Nuts
6. Pasta, bread, pizza
7. Whole milk
8. Dessert
9. Whole-milk dairy foods

This week's menu can contain food such as the following:

1. Protein shakes daily
2. Beef and chicken introduced slowly
3. Fish of any kind
4. Vegetables, soft
5. Sweet potatoes
6. Mashed potatoes
7. Baked potatoes
8. Cereal
9. Caffeine, a limited amount

If your surgeon gives approval for you to have snacks between meals, they may include foods such as the following:

1. Fresh fruit
2. ¼ of a baked sweet potato

3. ¼ cup of oatmeal

4. Hummus with boiled baby carrots

5. One hard-boiled egg

6. Hummus on rice crackers

Fifth Week to the Third Month

Continue to introduce food one by one and note how well you take each one. Eating something you don't tolerate well will give you constipation, upset stomach, or diarrhea. You will still eat things like cooked vegetables, canned or soft fruit, ground meat, and finely diced meat. Do not eat much of the solid or hard food yet. You must wait until the doctor clears you for those kinds of foods.

Eat three meals daily, still concentrating on protein intake. Drink lots of fluids throughout every day, but stop drinking 30 minutes before each meal. Try not to snack unless you have something nutritious, such as fruit, vegetables, or maybe a few nuts. Remember to take your vitamins. Be prepared for bad days so that you can cope. Find yourself an accountability partner in a support group or someone that you can call.

Third to Sixth Month

You likely have lost a very small amount of weight by now, and you probably feel glad you had the surgery! Your surgeon will approve solid foods for you now. You will feel full very fast now when you eat them. Chew them well. Eat slowly. You need to take it slowly because crunchy or spicy food may be difficult to tolerate at first. As before, you need to introduce one solid food at a time and see how well your system handles it. Write down any problems you experience. You should have a dietician that you meet with regularly by now. They will help you strategize blending your diet with those of your family and give you grocery shopping tips and tips for getting through holiday meals, etc.

You'll want to relax by this stage and start consuming things like Lactaid-free milk, almond milk, unsweetened coconut milk, blended Greek yogurt with no fruit chunks, unsweetened applesauce, cooked cereal such as oatmeal, grits or Cream of Wheat made with lactose-free milk, a blended soup made with lactose-free milk, blended fruit smoothies, and shakes. Do not combine food selections below at first in any one meal, but gradually try the following foods during this phase:

➢ Soft fruit

➢ Light white fish

➢ Crackers with peanut butter

➢ Cooked vegetables

➢ Yogurt with fruit

➢ Cooked eggs

➢ Blended soup

➢ Cottage cheese

➢ Oatmeal, grits, or Cream of Wheat

You can now tolerate meat, however, so you can test your level of tolerance and learn more about it. After all, you won't want to only consume breakfast food and sweet-tasting shakes for longer than you have to. Below, you can find sources of protein and also food from the various food groups that you ought to begin to consume during this phase.

CHAPTER 3: Early Post-Op Foods

The clear liquid that you need to take care of starts from the third day when you go home. During this early period, you will be able to drink only one ounce after every 15 minutes. The most important thing to practice is to drink slowly, as it hurts if you start dumping everything inside at once. After discharge from the hospital, you can start clear liquids. At this point, your home must have already been set up and ready for this clear liquid diet. Your kitchen should have the following things:

1. Protein shakes and powders in a variety of brands and flavors
2. High-protein soups
3. Broths, liquid-only soups, and low-fat cream soups
4. Yogurts, which should be non-fat plain Greek yogurt and other SF, non-fat flavors with fruits only on top
5. Bariatric liquid or chewable supplements as recommended by your dietician, including multivitamins, calcium citrate, probiotics, and Vitamin B12
6. Small spoons and dishes
7. All the sugar-free syrups
8. Herb and spice blends
9. Shake bottles

The post-op diet progresses from all the stages that go for about two months. This slow and gradual progression is created for the health and safety of the patient.

Dumping syndrome results when a lot of foods or beverages are dumped into the small intestine via the stomach due to overeating. When you instantly consume huge amounts of liquid or larger bites, it will strain the stomach and the intestines. Remember that now your stomach cannot hold the excess food for you; now, the food is directly going into the stomach. If you keep dumping the food in the intestine, it will fail to digest that food, which will lead to the following symptoms of discomfort, which are together known as the dumping syndrome.

Symptoms

1. Diarrhea
2. Pain
3. Nausea
4. Vomiting
5. Bloating
6. Abdominal cramps
7. Epigastric fullness
8. Sweating
9. Headache
10. Palpitations (rapid heart rate)
11. Lightheadedness
12. Flushing
13. A strong desire to lie down

Fortunately, dumping syndrome can be prevented by taking some basic measures. Mindful eating is one good method to keep yourself aware of the food portions you are consuming.

1. Avoid those foods and liquids that are high in sugar or saturated fats, as the intestine would fail to digest them quickly.

2. Do not drink all the nutrients through your drinks; try using a straw to take small sips.

3. Don't eat full-fat dairy products. Low-fat dairy is typically fine.

4. Do not consume cookies, juices, ice cream, rice, pasta, bread, crackers, pizza, and similar food items.

5. Avoid high-fat meats, hot dogs, pork sausage, burgers, bacon, pepperoni, etc.

Liquid Diet

The liquid diet comes with its own requirements and requisites. This liquid diet is not like the other diets; in the liquid gastric diet, it is important to control the caloric intake as well as the amount of the liquid. Determine the amount initially; it requires a small number of liquids to start with. About four ounces per 15 minutes, then switch to ten ounces, and then finally to 40 ounces. The liquid is essential to keep yourself hydrated all the time. Once the stomach is healed and there are no risks of staple line leakage, you can start consuming it in a large amount. Regulate food intake, and knowing what types of liquid you are consuming is also important to understand. Low caloric liquids should be added to clear liquid diets.

Many people experience a change in taste preferences after surgery. It is recommended to have several different flavors and brands in your hand in case this also happens to you; then, you will have an extra option to avail yourself. Get a variety of protein shakes and powders to determine the ones you like best.

Chocolate, vanilla, unflavored protein powder, and chicken soup can be flavored to your liking. After surgery, your nutritional needs also change as the body adapts to the new lifestyle, so you should start reading the product labels of food products to ensure that you are consuming all the right products to meet your protein requirements. Shakes with insufficient protein and high calories can also lead to dumping syndrome, especially when the sugar content is too high.

1. Yogurt: Non-fat, plain Greek yogurt with added sugar or fruit.

2. Soups and broths with protein powders without any flavors added.

3. Buy several different flavors and seasonings to increase variety.

4. High-protein soups like beef, chicken, or tomato protein soup.

5. Liquid-only soups, including tomato, squash, or carrot soup.

6. There are many unflavored protein powders available. Make sure to keep these powders at a temperature under 140 degrees.

7. Stir in flavored protein powders, sugar-free syrups, stevia-flavored drops to add a variety of flavors.

8. Low-fat cream soups like creams of chicken, mushroom, broccoli, strained.

9. Broth, bouillon, or bone broth are clear liquids.

10. No high-fat cream soups; avoid noodles or rice soups.

11. No chili, bean, or lentil soups.

It is important to follow the diet-specific guidelines that your bariatric dietitian has recommended to you after knowing your health conditions. You can find a lot of relevant information about post-op bariatric diets, but these guidelines are general and are advised to all. However, each person must follow those rules in light of their own body needs and requirements.

CHAPTER 4: Recipes for Recovery
STAGE 1: CLEAR LIQUID RECIPES

Apple Juice

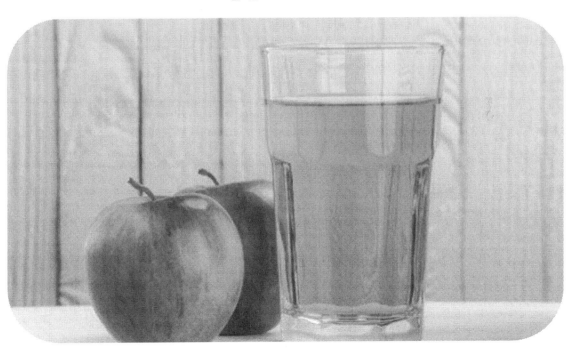

Ingredients

- ➤ 5 large apples, cored and chopped
- ➤ 1 small lemon
- ➤ 1 cup filtered water

How to Prepare

1. In a high-powered blender, add apples, lemon, and water, and pulse until well blended.
2. Through a cheesecloth-lined strainer, strain the juice and transfer into 2 glasses.
3. Serve immediately.

Preparation time: 10 minutes
Total time: 10 minutes
Servings: 2

Nutritional Values

- ➤ *Calories 292*
- ➤ *Total Fat 1 g*
- ➤ *Saturated Fat 0 g*
- ➤ *Cholesterol 0 mg*
- ➤ *Sodium 5 mg*
- ➤ *Total Carbs 77.7 g*
- ➤ *Fiber 13.7 g*
- ➤ *Sugar 58.2 g*
- ➤ *Protein 1.6 g*

Citrus Detox Water

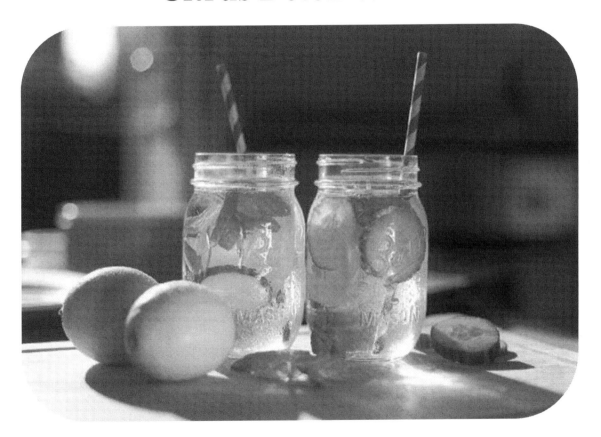

Ingredients

- ➢ 1 lime, sliced
- ➢ 1 lemon, sliced
- ➢ 1 cucumber, sliced
- ➢ 2 tablespoons fresh mint leaves

> 6 cups filtered water

How to Prepare

1. In a large glass jar, place fruit, cucumber, and mint leaves, and pour water on top.

2. Cover the jar with a lid tightly and refrigerate for about 2–4 hours before serving.

Preparation time: 10 minutes

Total time: 10 minutes

Servings: 3

Nutritional Values

> *Calories 20*
> *Total Fat 0.2 g*
> *Saturated Fat 0.1 g*
> *Cholesterol 0 mg*
> *Sodium 3 mg*
> *Total Carbs 5 g*
> *Fiber 1 g*
> *Sugar 1.9 g*
> *Protein 0.9 g*

Lemonade

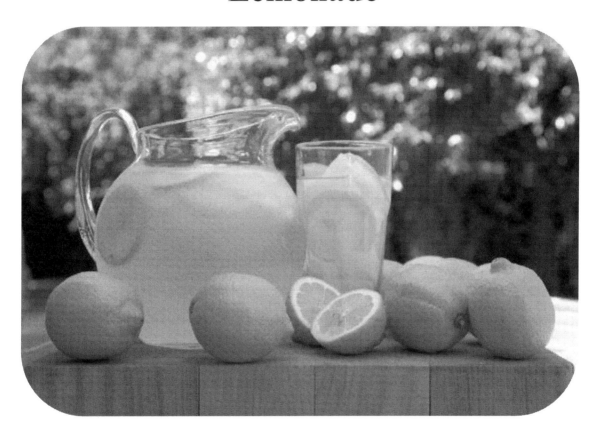

Ingredients

- ¾ cup fresh lemon juice
- 8–10 drops liquid stevia
- 3½ cups cold sparkling water
- Ice cubes, as needed

How to Prepare

1. In a pitcher, place lemon juice and stevia, and stir to combine.

2. Add the water and fill the pitcher with ice.

3. Serve chilled.

Preparation time: 10 minutes
Total time: 10 minutes
Servings: 4

Nutritional Values

➢ *Calories 11*
➢ *Total Fat 0.4 g*
➢ *Saturated Fat 0.4 g*
➢ *Cholesterol 0 mg*
➢ *Sodium 9 mg*
➢ *Total Carbs 1 g*
➢ *Fiber 0.2 g*
➢ *Sugar 1 g*
➢ *Protein 0.4 g*

Black Tea

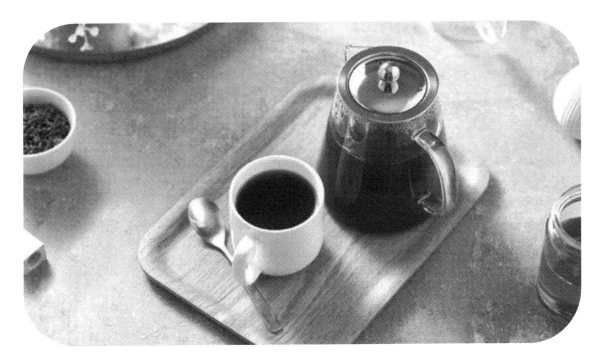

Ingredients

- ➤ 2 cups water
- ➤ 1–2 teaspoons decaffeinated loose leaf black tea
- ➤ 2–3 drops liquid stevia

How to Prepare

1. In a small saucepan, add water over medium heat and bring to a rolling boil.

2. Stir in in tea and turn off the heat.

3. Immediately, cover the pan for 2 minutes.

4. Stir in stevia and serve hot.

Preparation time: 5 minutes

Cooking time: 5 minutes

Total time: 10 minutes

Servings: 2

Nutritional Values

➢ *Calories 1*

➢ *Total Fat 0 g*

➢ *Saturated Fat 0 g*

➢ *Cholesterol 0 mg*

➢ *Sodium 0 mg*

➢ *Total Carbs 0.1 g*

➢ *Fiber 0 g*

➢ *Sugar 0 g*

➢ *Protein 0.1 g*

Lemon Ginger Tea

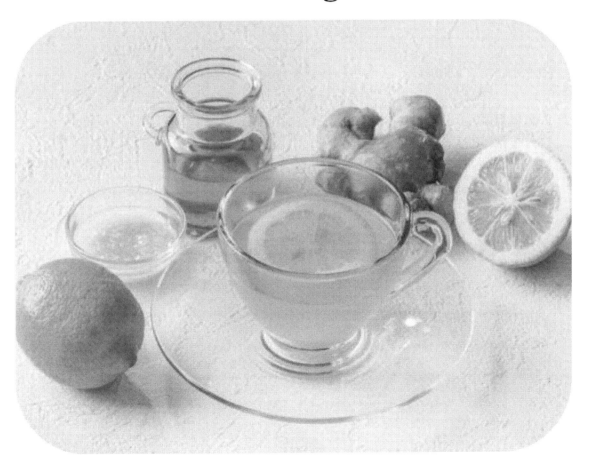

Ingredients

- ➤ 6 cups water
- ➤ ½ of lemon, seeded and chopped roughly
- ➤ 1 (1-inch) piece fresh ginger, chopped

49

- ➤ 2 tablespoons maple syrup
- ➤ Pinch of ground turmeric
- ➤ Pinch of ground cinnamon

How to Prepare

1. In a saucepan, add all ingredients over medium-high heat and bring to a boil.
2. Adjust the heat to medium-low and simmer for about 10–12 minutes.
3. Strain into cups and serve hot.

Preparation time: 10 minutes
Cooking time: 15 minutes
Total time: 25 minutes
Servings: 4

Nutritional Values

- ➤ *Calories 32*
- ➤ *Total Fat 0.1 g*
- ➤ *Saturated Fat 0 g*
- ➤ *Cholesterol 0 mg*
- ➤ *Sodium 1 mg*
- ➤ *Total Carbs 8 g*
- ➤ *Fiber 0.3 g*
- ➤ *Sugar 6.1 g*
- ➤ *Protein 0.2 g*

Black Coffee

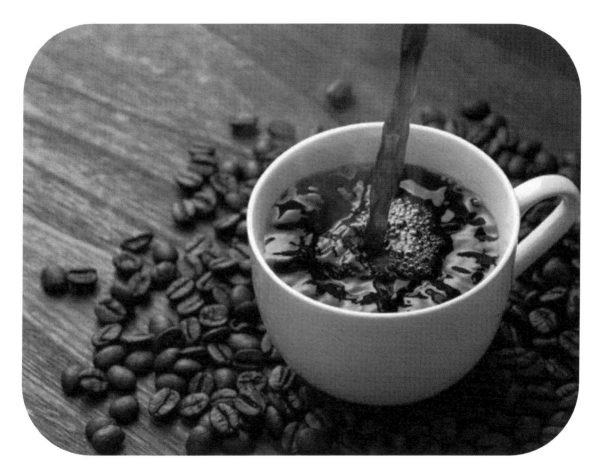

Ingredients

➢ ½ tablespoon decaffeinated instant coffee powder

➢ 1–2 drops liquid stevia

➢ 1 cup boiling water

How to Prepare

1. In a mug, add coffee, stevia, and boiling water, and stir until well combined.
2. Serve hot.

Preparation time: 6 minutes
Total time: 5 minutes
Servings: 1

Nutritional Values

➢ *Calories 3*
➢ *Total Fat 0 g*
➢ *Saturated Fat 0 g*
➢ *Cholesterol 0 mg*
➢ *Sodium 1 mg*
➢ *Total Carbs 0.6 g*
➢ *Fiber 0 g*
➢ *Sugar 0 g*
➢ *Protein 0.2 g*

Chicken Broth

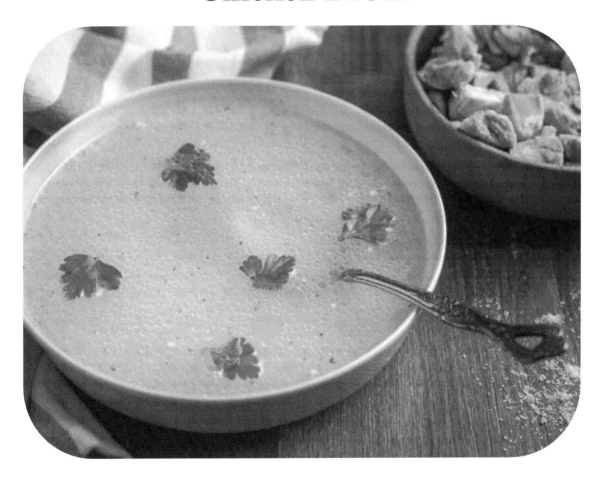

Ingredients

- ➢ 1 (3-pound) chicken, cut into pieces
- ➢ 5–6 medium carrots, peeled and cut into pieces
- ➢ 4 celery stalks with leaves, cut into 2-inch pieces

- ➢ 6 fresh thyme sprigs
- ➢ 6 fresh parsley sprigs
- ➢ Salt, as needed
- ➢ 9 cups cold water

How to Prepare

1. In a saucepan, add all the ingredients over medium-high heat and bring to a boil.
2. Now adjust the heat to medium-low and simmer, covered for about 2 hours, skimming the foam from the surface occasionally.
3. Through a fine-mesh sieve, strain the broth into a large bowl.
4. Serve hot.

Preparation time: 15 minutes
Cooking time: 2 hours 5 minutes
Total time: 2 hours 20 minutes
Servings: 8

Nutritional Values

- ➢ *Calories 276*
- ➢ *Total Fat 5.2 g*
- ➢ *Saturated Fat 1.5 g*
- ➢ *Cholesterol 131 mg*
- ➢ *Sodium 161 mg*
- ➢ *Total Carbs 4.4 g*
- ➢ *Fiber 1.3 g*
- ➢ *Sugar 2 g*
- ➢ *Protein 49.7 g*

Peach Gelatin

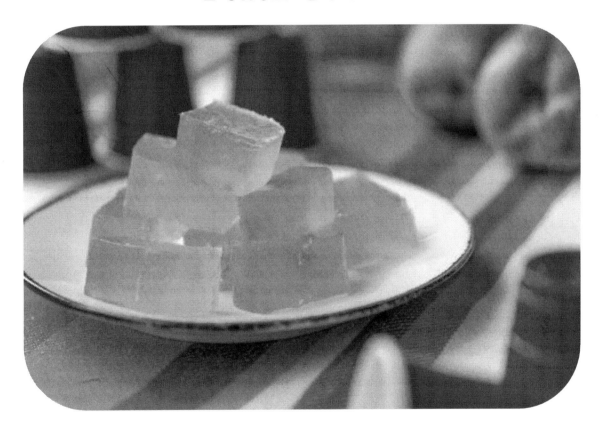

Ingredients

- ➢ 2 tablespoons grass-fed gelatin powder
- ➢ 4 cups fresh peach juice, divided
- ➢ 2 tablespoons maple syrup

How to Prepare

1. In a bowl, soak the gelatin in ½ cup of juice. Set aside for about 5 minutes.

2. In a medium pan, add the remaining juice over medium heat and bring to a gentle boil.

3. Remove from the heat and stir in maple syrup.

4. Add the gelatin mixture and stir until dissolved.

5. Transfer the mixture into a large baking dish and refrigerate until set completely before serving.

Preparation time: 10 minutes

Cooking time: 5 minutes

Total time: 15 minutes

Servings: 10

Nutritional Values

➢ *Calories 65*

➢ *Total Fat 0 g*

➢ *Saturated Fat 0 g*

➢ *Cholesterol 0 mg*

➢ *Sodium 8 mg*

➢ *Total Carbs 14.7 g*

➢ *Fiber 0 g*

➢ *Sugar 13.2 g*

➢ *Protein 1.8 g*

Lemon Gelatin

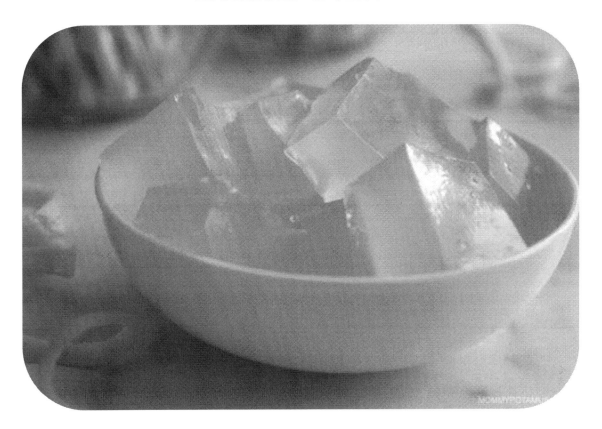

Ingredients

- ➢ 3 tablespoons grass-fed gelatin powder
- ➢ 3 cups cold water, divided
- ➢ 1½ cups boiling water
- ➢ 1 cup plus 2 tablespoons freshly squeezed lemon juice
- ➢ 2 teaspoons stevia extract

How to Prepare

1. In a bowl, soak the gelatin in 1½ cups of cold water. Set aside for about 5 minutes.

2. Add the boiling water and stir until gelatin is dissolved.

3. Add the remaining cold water, lemon juice, and stevia extract, and stir until dissolved completely.

4. Divide the mixture into 2 baking dishes and refrigerate until set before serving.

Preparation time: 10 minutes

Total time: 10 minutes

Servings: 8

Nutritional Values

- ➤ *Calories 21*
- ➤ *Total Fat 0.3 g*
- ➤ *Saturated Fat 0.3 g*
- ➤ *Cholesterol 0 mg*
- ➤ *Sodium 17 mg*
- ➤ *Total Carbs 0.7 g*
- ➤ *Fiber 0.1 g*
- ➤ *Sugar 0.7 g*
- ➤ *Protein 3.7 g*

Cucumber & Kiwi Popsicles

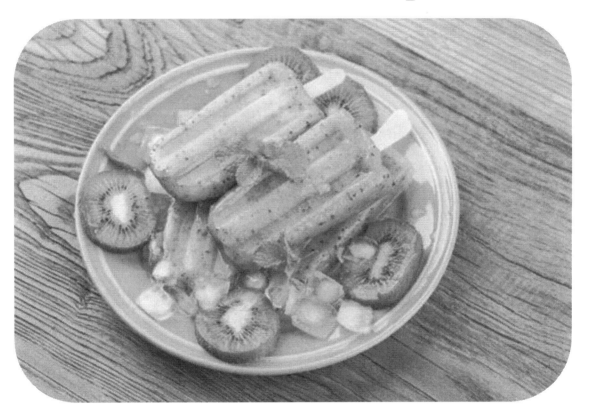

Ingredients

- ➤ 1 pound cucumbers, chopped
- ➤ 4 kiwis, peeled
- ➤ 1¼ cups fresh mint leaves
- ➤ ½ cup fresh lime juice

- ➤ ¼ cup maple syrup
- ➤ 1¼ cups water

How to Prepare

1. In a high-powered blender, put all ingredients and pulse until smooth.
2. Transfer the kiwi mixture into the Popsicle molds and freeze for 4 hours before serving.

Preparation time: 15 minutes

Total time: 15 minutes

Servings: 8

Nutritional Values

- ➤ *Calories 65*
- ➤ *Total Fat 0.4 g*
- ➤ *Saturated Fat 0.1 g*
- ➤ *Cholesterol 0 mg*
- ➤ *Sodium 7 mg*
- ➤ *Total Carbs 15.6 g*
- ➤ *Fiber 2.4 g*
- ➤ *Sugar 10.2 g*
- ➤ *Protein 1.3 g*

STAGE 2: PUREED FOOD RECIPES

Protein Smoothie

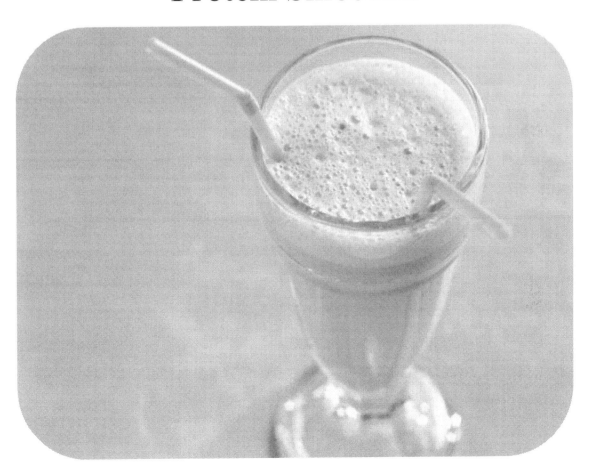

Ingredients

➢ ½ cup unsweetened protein powder

➢ 1 tablespoon almond butter

➢ 2 teaspoons vanilla extract

➢ 6–8 drops liquid stevia

➢ 1½ cups unsweetened almond milk

➢ ¼ cup ice cubes

How to Prepare

1. In a high-powered blender, put all ingredients and pulse until creamy.

2. Place the smoothie into two serving glasses and serve immediately.

Preparation time: 10 minutes

Total time: 10 minutes

Servings: 2

Nutritional Values

➢ *Calories 198*

➢ *Total Fat 8.4 g*

➢ *Saturated Fat 0.9 g*

➢ *Cholesterol 24 mg*

➢ *Sodium 185 mg*

➢ *Total Carbs 5.4 g*

➢ *Fiber 1.6 g*

➢ *Sugar 2.1 g*

➢ *Protein 24.5 g*

Egg Yogurt Salad

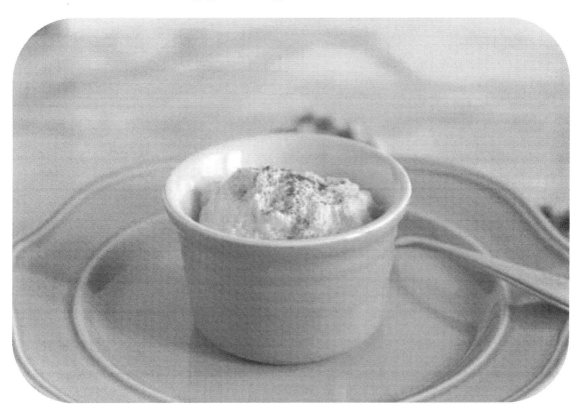

Ingredients

- ➤ 2 hard-boiled eggs, peeled and sliced
- ➤ 1 tablespoon plain Greek-style yogurt
- ➤ 1 tablespoon low-fat mayonnaise
- ➤ Salt and ground black pepper, as needed

How to Prepare

1. Place the egg slices in a food processor and pulse until finely chopped.

2. Add the remaining ingredients and pulse until smooth.

Preparation time: 10 minutes

Total time: 10 minutes

Servings: 2

Nutritional Values

- ➤ *Calories 97*
- ➤ *Total Fat 6.9 g*
- ➤ *Saturated Fat 1.8 g*
- ➤ *Cholesterol 166 mg*
- ➤ *Sodium 197 mg*
- ➤ *Total Carbs 2.6 g*
- ➤ *Fiber 0 g*
- ➤ *Sugar 1.4 g*
- ➤ *Protein 6.1 g*

Chicken & Tomato Sauce Puree

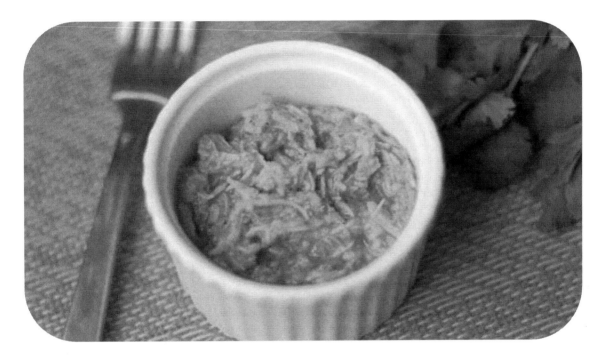

Ingredients

- ¼ cup canned chicken
- 1½ tablespoons tomato sauce
- 1/8 teaspoon salt
- 1/8 teaspoon ground black pepper
- 1 teaspoon Italian seasoning

How to Prepare

1. In a high-powered blender, put all ingredients and pulse until smooth.

2. Transfer the mixture into a microwave-safe bowl and microwave for about 30 seconds.

3. Serve immediately.

Preparation time: 10 minutes

Cooking time ½ minute

Total time: 10½ minutes

Servings: 1

Nutritional Values

- ➢ *Calories 73*
- ➢ *Total Fat 2.5 g*
- ➢ *Saturated Fat 0.5 g*
- ➢ *Cholesterol 30 mg*
- ➢ *Sodium 435 mg*
- ➢ *Total Carbs 1.9 g*
- ➢ *Fiber 0.4 g*
- ➢ *Sugar 1.4 g*
- ➢ *Protein 10.5 g*

Chicken Liver Pate

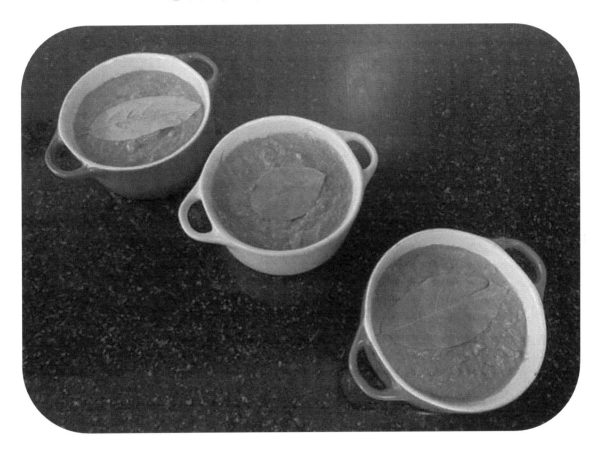

Ingredients

➢ 1 tablespoon low-fat spread

➢ 1 red onion, peeled and finely chopped

➢ 1 garlic clove, crushed

- ➤ ½ pound chicken livers, washed and trimmed
- ➤ 2 teaspoon concentrated tomato puree
- ➤ Salt and ground black pepper, as needed
- ➤ 2 tablespoons fat-free fromage frais
- ➤ 3 tablespoons low-fat butter, melted

How to Prepare

1. In a non-stick frying pan, melt the spread over medium-low heat and sauté the onion and garlic for about 5 minutes or until softened.
2. Add the chicken livers and cook for about 5–8 minutes or until cooked through.
3. Stir in the tomato puree, salt, and black pepper, and remove from the heat.
4. Set aside to cool.
5. Place the chicken liver mixture and fromage frais into a food processor and pulse until smooth.
6. Transfer the mixture to a serving bowl.
7. With a plastic wrap, cover the dish and refrigerate for at least 2 hours before serving.

Preparation time: 15 minutes
Cooking time: 13 minutes
Total time: 28 minutes
Servings: 4

Nutritional Values
- ➤ *Calories 178*
- ➤ *Total Fat 9.1 g*
- ➤ *Saturated Fat 2 g*

- Cholesterol 319 mg
- Sodium 114 mg
- Total Carbs 7.6 g
- Fiber 1.4 g
- Sugar 2.3 g
- Protein 16.7 g

Smoked Salmon Pate

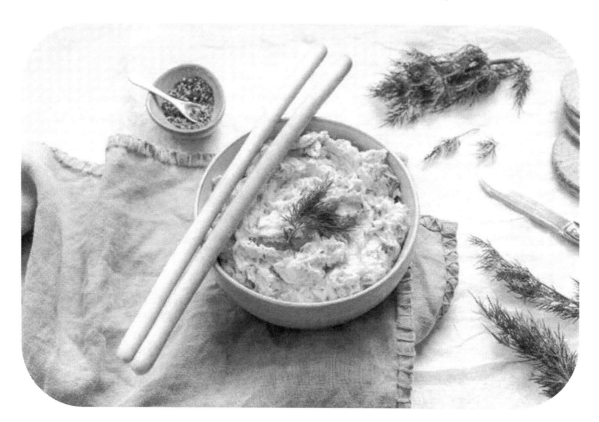

Ingredients

➢ 2½ ounces fresh smoked salmon

➢ 2 tablespoons fat-free plain Greek yogurt

➢ ½ teaspoon dried dill

➢ 1 tablespoon fresh lemon juice

- 1/8 teaspoon salt
- 1/8 teaspoon ground black pepper

How to Prepare

1. In a high-powered food processor, add all ingredients and pulse until smooth.
2. Serve immediately.

Preparation time: 10 minutes
Total time: 10 minutes
Servings: 1

Nutritional Values

- *Calories 101*
- *Total Fat 3.2 g*
- *Saturated Fat 0.8 g*
- *Cholesterol 18 mg*
- *Sodium 900 mg*
- *Total Carbs 2.8 g*
- *Fiber 0.2 g*
- *Sugar 1.6 g*
- *Protein 14.5 g*

Tuna Yogurt Puree

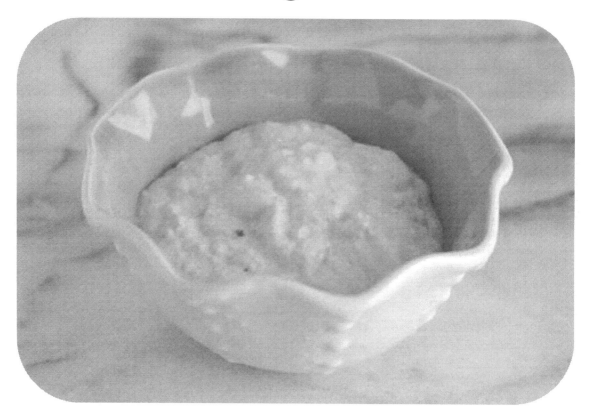

Ingredients

➢ 1 (6-ounce) can water-packed tuna, drained

➢ 2 teaspoons relish

➢ 2 tablespoons low-fat mayonnaise

➢ 2 tablespoons plain Greek yogurt

➤ Salt and ground black pepper, as needed

How to Prepare

1. In a high-powered food processor, add all ingredients and pulse until smooth.
2. Serve immediately.

Preparation time: 10 minutes
Total time: 10 minutes
Servings: 4

Nutritional Values

➤ *Calories 87*
➤ *Total Fat 2.9 g*
➤ *Saturated Fat 0.5 g*
➤ *Cholesterol 15 mg*
➤ *Sodium 138 mg*
➤ *Total Carbs 3.2 g*
➤ *Fiber 0 g*
➤ *Sugar 1.7 g*
➤ *Protein 11.4 g*

Shrimp Puree

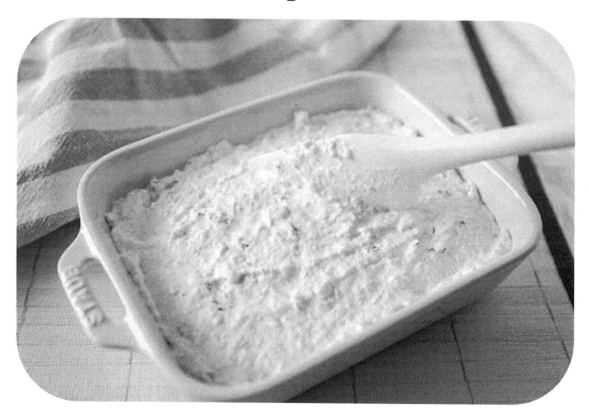

Ingredients

- ➤ 16 ounces cooked shrimp
- ➤ 8 ounce low-fat cream cheese, softened
- ➤ ½ cup low-fat plain Greek yogurt
- ➤ 8 ounces sugar-free cocktail sauce

How to Prepare

1. In a high-powered food processor, add all ingredients and pulse until smooth.

2. Serve immediately.

Preparation time: 10 minutes

Total time: 20 minutes

Servings: 10

Nutritional Values

- ➢ *Calories 190*
- ➢ *Total Fat 8.8 g*
- ➢ *Saturated Fat 5.3 g*
- ➢ *Cholesterol 121 mg*
- ➢ *Sodium 626 mg*
- ➢ *Total Carbs 11.8 g*
- ➢ *Fiber 0.8 g*
- ➢ *Sugar 4.1 g*
- ➢ *Protein 13.5 g*

Black Beans Puree

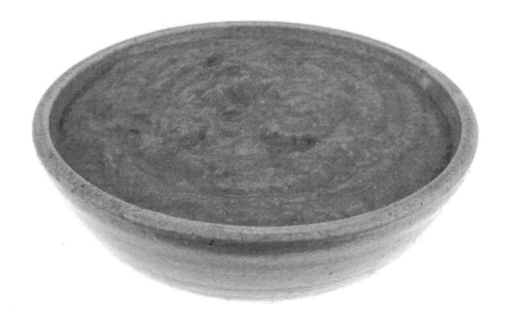

Ingredients

- ➤ ¼ cup canned black beans, rinsed
- ➤ ½ tablespoon fresh lime juice
- ➤ ½ tablespoon juice from jarred jalapeños
- ➤ ¼ cup low-fat chicken broth

How to Prepare

1. Place the black beans, lime juice, and juice from jarred jalapeños in a small saucepan over medium heat, and stir to combine.

2. Place the saucepan of beans mixture over medium heat and cook for about 3–5 minutes, stirring frequently.

3. Stir in the chicken broth and remove from the heat.

4. In a blender, add the beans mixture and pulse until smooth.

5. Set aside to cool slightly.

6. Add the protein powder and stir until well combined.

7. Serve immediately.

Preparation time: 10 minutes
Cooking time: 5 minutes
Total time: 15 minutes
Servings: 1

Nutritional Values

- ➢ *Calories 175*
- ➢ *Total Fat 1 g*
- ➢ *Saturated Fat 0.3 g*
- ➢ *Cholesterol 0 mg*
- ➢ *Sodium 35 mg*
- ➢ *Total Carbs 30.3 g*
- ➢ *Fiber 7.4 g*
- ➢ *Sugar 1 g*
- ➢ *Protein 11.7 g*

Ranch Cottage Cheese

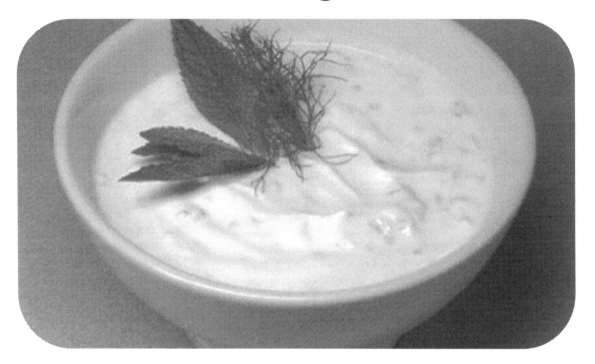

Ingredients

- ➢ 4 ounces low-fat cottage cheese with chives
- ➢ 2 teaspoons dry ranch dressing mix
- ➢ Pinch of ground black pepper

How to Prepare

1. In a bowl, put all ingredients and stir to combine.

2. Serve immediately.

Preparation time: 5 minutes
Total time: 5 minutes
Servings: 2

Nutritional Values

➢ *Calories 53*
➢ *Total Fat 1.1 g*
➢ *Saturated Fat 0.7 g*
➢ *Cholesterol 5 mg*
➢ *Sodium 258 mg*
➢ *Total Carbs 2.4 g*
➢ *Fiber 0 g*
➢ *Sugar 0.3 g*
➢ *Protein 7.9 g*

Lemon Ricotta Cream

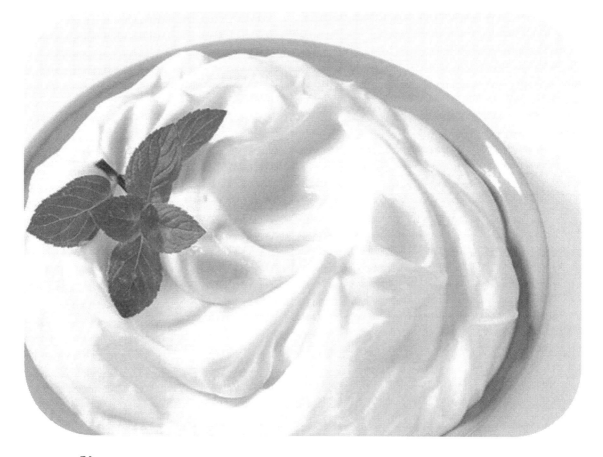

Ingredients

➢ 1 (15-ounce) container low-fat ricotta cheese

➢ 1 teaspoon lemon zest, grated

➢ 1–2 teaspoons lemon extract

- ➤ 1½ teaspoons vanilla extract
- ➤ 4 packets Splenda

How to Prepare

1. Put all the ingredients in a high-powered food processor and pulse until smooth.
2. Serve immediately.

Preparation time: 10 minutes
Total time: 10 minutes
Servings: 3

Nutritional Values

- ➤ *Calories 220*
- ➤ *Total Fat 11.2 g*
- ➤ *Saturated Fat 7 g*
- ➤ *Cholesterol 44 mg*
- ➤ *Sodium 177 mg*
- ➤ *Total Carbs 11.6 g*
- ➤ *Fiber 0 g*
- ➤ *Sugar 4.7 g*
- ➤ *Protein 0.2 g*

STAGE 3: SOFT FOOD RECIPES

Oats & Mango Smoothie

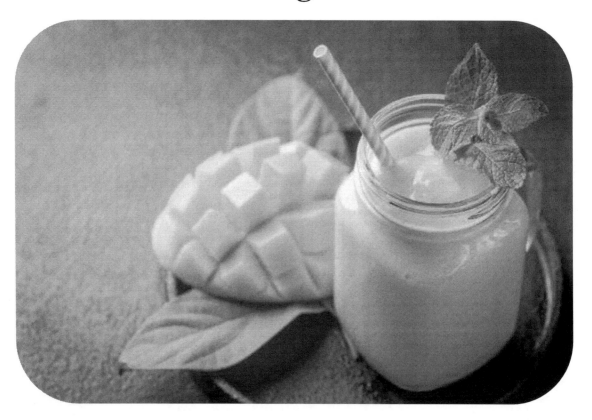

Ingredients
 ➢ 1 cup mango; peeled, pitted, and chopped

- ¼ cup quick oats
- ¾ cup low-fat cottage cheese
- 1 tablespoon maple syrup
- 1½ cups unsweetened almond milk
- ¼ cup ice cubes

How to Prepare

1. In a high-powered blender, put all ingredients and pulse until creamy.
2. Place the smoothie into two serving glasses and serve.

Preparation time: 10 minutes

Total time: 10 minutes

Servings: 2

Nutritional Values

- *Calories 221*
- *Total Fat 5.3 g*
- *Saturated Fat 1.5 g*
- *Cholesterol 7 mg*
- *Sodium 481 mg*
- *Total Carbs 30.6 g*
- *Fiber 3.1 g*
- *Sugar 17.6 g*
- *Protein 4.1 g*

Strawberry Smoothie Bowl

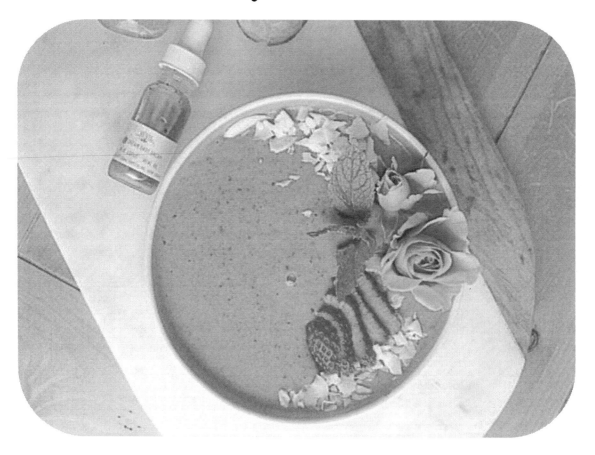

Ingredients

➢ 2 cups frozen strawberries

➢ ½ cup unsweetened almond milk

➢ ¼ cup fat-free plain Greek yogurt

➤ 1 tablespoon unsweetened whey protein powder

How to Prepare

1. In a high-powdered blender, add frozen strawberries and pulse for about 1 minute.
2. Add the almond milk, yogurt, and protein powder, and pulse until desired consistency is achieved.
3. Transfer the mixture into 2 serving bowls evenly.
4. Serve immediately with your favorite topping.

Preparation time: 10 minutes
Total time: 10 minutes
Servings: 2

Nutritional Values

➤ *Calories 83*
➤ *Total Fat 1.5 g*
➤ *Saturated Fat 0.1 g*
➤ *Cholesterol 1 mg*
➤ *Sodium 99 mg*
➤ *Total Carbs 13.7 g*
➤ *Fiber 3.1 g*
➤ *Sugar 7.1 g*
➤ *Protein 5.4 g*

Spinach Smoothie Bowl

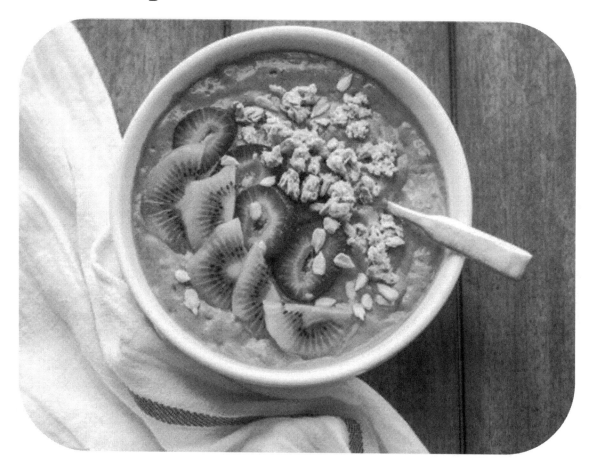

Ingredients

➢ 2 cups fresh spinach

➢ 1 medium avocado; peeled, pitted, and chopped roughly

➢ 2 scoops unsweetened protein powder

- ➤ 3 tablespoons maple syrup
- ➤ 2 tablespoons fresh lemon juice
- ➤ 1 cup unsweetened almond milk
- ➤ ¼ cup ice cubes

How to Prepare

1. In a high-powdered blender, put all the ingredients and pulse until smooth.
2. Transfer into 2 serving bowls and serve with your favorite topping.

Preparation time: 10 minutes

Total time: 10 minutes

Servings: 2

Nutritional Values

- ➤ *Calories 314*
- ➤ *Total Fat 22.7 g*
- ➤ *Saturated Fat 4.4 g*
- ➤ *Cholesterol 0 mg*
- ➤ *Sodium 390 mg*
- ➤ *Total Carbs 31.2 g*
- ➤ *Fiber 8 g*
- ➤ *Sugar 18.8 g*
- ➤ *Protein 28.7 g*

Avocado & Egg Salad

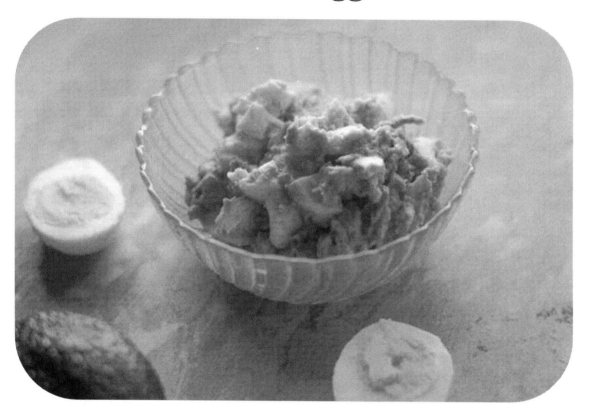

Ingredients
➤ 6 hard-boiled eggs, peeled

➤ 2 ripe avocados, peeled and pitted

➤ 1 tablespoon fresh lemon juice

➤ 2 celery stalks, chopped

- ½ of purple onion, chopped
- ½ teaspoon Dijon mustard
- ½ teaspoon salt
- Pinch of ground black pepper

How to Prepare

1. Cut each boiled egg in half and transfer the yolks into a small bowl.
2. Cut the whites into small pieces and transfer into another bowl.
3. In the bowl of egg yolks, add 1 avocado, and with a fork, mash until well combined.
4. Add the mustard, lemon juice, salt, and black pepper, and mix well. Set aside.
5. Chop the remaining avocado and transfer into the bowl of egg whites.
6. Add the celery and onion whites and mix well.
7. Add the egg yolk mixture and gently stir to combine.
8. Refrigerate to chill for about 2 hours before serving.

Preparation time: 15 minutes
Total time: 15 minutes
Servings: 4

Nutritional Values

- *Calories 308*
- *Total Fat 26.2 g*
- *Saturated Fat 6.2 g*
- *Cholesterol 246 mg*
- *Sodium 404 mg*

- *Total Carbs 10.8 g*
- *Fiber 7.2 g*
- *Sugar 1.8 g*
- *Protein 10.5 g*

Chicken-Stuffed Avocado

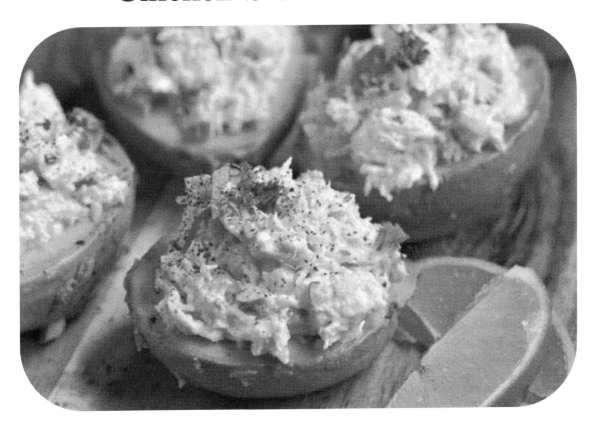

Ingredients

➢ ½ cup cooked chicken, shredded

➢ 1 avocado, halved and pitted

➢ 1 tablespoon fresh lime juice

➢ ¼ cup yellow onion, chopped finely

➢ ¼ cup fat-free plain Greek yogurt

- ➤ 1 teaspoon Dijon mustard
- ➤ Pinch of cayenne pepper
- ➤ Salt and ground black pepper, as needed

How to Prepare

1. With a small scooper, scoop out the flesh from middle of each avocado half and transfer into a bowl.
2. Add the lime juice and mash until well combined.
3. Add remaining ingredients and stir to combine.
4. Divide the chicken mixture in avocado halves evenly and serve immediately.

Preparation time: 15 minutes
Total time: 15 minutes
Servings: 2

Nutritional Values

- ➤ *Calories 280*
- ➤ *Total Fat 20.8 g*
- ➤ *Saturated Fat 4.4 g*
- ➤ *Cholesterol 28 mg*
- ➤ *Sodium 156 mg*
- ➤ *Total Carbs 12.4 g*
- ➤ *Fiber 7.2 g*
- ➤ *Sugar 1.1 g*
- ➤ *Protein 13.6 g*

Ricotta & Parmesan Bake

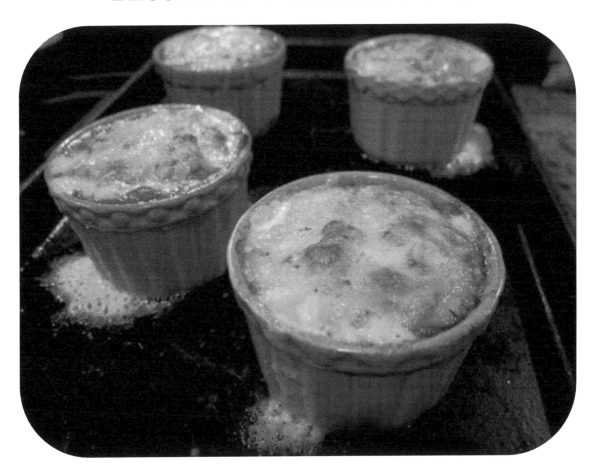

Ingredients

➢ 15 ounces part-skim ricotta cheese

➢ 1/3 cup low-fat Parmesan cheese, grated

➢ 1/8 teaspoon dried basil

- ➤ 1/8 teaspoon garlic powder
- ➤ Pinch of salt and ground black pepper
- ➤ 5 tablespoons sugar-free marinara sauce

How to Prepare

1. Preheat your oven to 350°F.
2. Grease 5 ramekins.
3. Arrange the ramekins onto a baking sheet.
4. In a bowl, put the ricotta cheese, Parmesan cheese, basil, garlic powder, salt, and black pepper, and mix well.
5. Divide the mixture into the prepared ramekins evenly and top each with 1 tablespoon of marinara sauce.
6. Arrange the ramekins onto a baking sheet.
7. Bake for approximately 20 minutes.
8. Serve warm.

Preparation time: 10 minutes
Cooking time: 20 minutes
Total time: 30 minutes
Servings: 5

Nutritional Values

- ➤ *Calories 139*
- ➤ *Total Fat 8.1 g*
- ➤ *Saturated Fat 5.1 g*
- ➤ *Cholesterol 32 mg*

- Sodium 255 mg
- Total Carbs 5.3 g
- Fiber 0.3 g
- Sugar 0.8 g
- Protein 11.3 g

3-Cheese Casserole

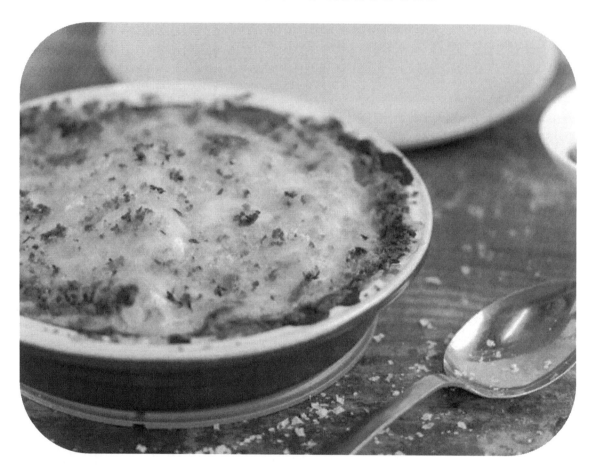

Ingredients

➢ 8 ounces part-skim ricotta cheese

➢ ½ cup low-fat Parmesan cheese, grated

- ➤ 1 large egg, beaten
- ➤ 1 teaspoon Italian seasoning
- ➤ Salt and ground black pepper, as needed
- ➤ ½ cup sugar-free marinara sauce
- ➤ ½ cup part-skim mozzarella cheese, shredded

How to Prepare

1. Preheat your oven to 350°F.
2. In a bowl, put the ricotta cheese, Parmesan cheese, egg, Italian seasoning, salt, and black pepper, and mix well.
3. Place the mixture into a baking dish and top each with 1 tablespoon of marinara sauce, followed by the mozzarella cheese.
4. Bake for approximately 20–25 minutes.
5. Serve warm.

Preparation time: 10 minutes
Cooking time: 25 minutes
Total time: 35 minutes
Servings: 8

Nutritional Values

- ➤ *Calories 85*
- ➤ *Total Fat 5 g*
- ➤ *Saturated Fat 2.8 g*
- ➤ *Cholesterol 39 mg*
- ➤ *Sodium 234 mg*

- ➤ *Total Carbs 3.9 g*
- ➤ *Fiber 0.4 g*
- ➤ *Sugar 1.6 g*
- ➤ *Protein 6.1 g*

Cauliflower Bake

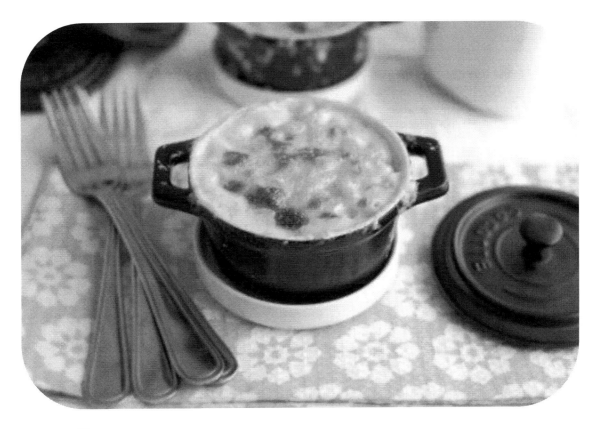

Ingredients

- ➤ 1 head cauliflower chopped (florets removed)
- ➤ ¼ cup heavy cream
- ➤ 1 tablespoon butter

> Salt and ground black pepper, as needed

> 3 tablespoons low-fat cheddar cheese, shredded

How to Prepare

1. Preheat your oven to broiler.

2. Lightly grease 3 ramekins.

3. In a pan of the boiling water, cook the cauliflower for about 4–5 minutes.

4. Through a colander, drain the cauliflower well.

5. In a bowl, place the cauliflower and with an immersion blender, blend until pureed.

6. Add the heavy cream, butter, salt, and black pepper, and mix well.

7. Divide the mixture into the prepared ramekins evenly and top each with cheddar cheese.

8. Arrange the ramekins onto a baking sheet.

9. Broil for approximately 3–5 minutes or until cheese is bubbly.

10. Serve warm.

Preparation time: 15 minutes

Cooking time: 10 minutes

Total time: 25 minutes

Servings: 3

Nutritional Values

> *Calories 119*

> *Total Fat 10 g*

> *Saturated Fat 6.2 g*

- ➤ *Cholesterol 31 mg*
- ➤ *Sodium 152 mg*
- ➤ *Total Carbs 5.1 g*
- ➤ *Fiber 2.2 g*
- ➤ *Sugar 2.2 g*
- ➤ *Protein 3.8 g*

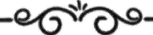

Tomato Soup

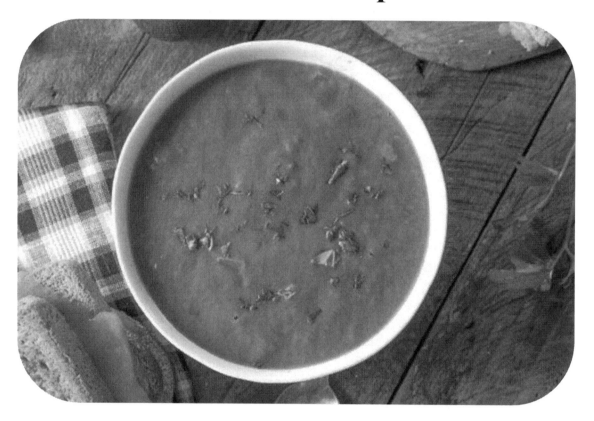

Ingredients
- ➢ 2 tablespoons olive oil
- ➢ 1 cup red onion, chopped
- ➢ 2¼ cups fresh tomatoes, chopped finely
- ➢ ½ teaspoon dried thyme, crushed

- ➤ 3 cups filtered water
- ➤ ¼ cup fresh basil leaves, chopped
- ➤ Salt and ground black pepper, as needed

How to Prepare

1. In a soup pan, heat the oil over medium heat and sauté onion for about 4–5 minutes.
2. Add the tomatoes, thyme, and water, and bring to a boil.
3. Now adjust the heat to low and simmer, covered for about 15 minutes.
4. Remove from the heat and set aside to cool slightly.
5. In a blender, add soup in batches and pulse until smooth.
6. Return the soup in the same pan over medium heat.
7. Stir in basil and cook for about 3–4 minutes.
8. Season with salt and black pepper and serve hot.

Preparation time: 10 minutes
Cooking time: 20 minutes
Total time: 30 minutes
Servings: 4

Nutritional Values

- ➤ *Calories 90*
- ➤ *Total Fat 7.3 g*
- ➤ *Saturated Fat 1 g*
- ➤ *Cholesterol 0 mg*
- ➤ *Sodium 45 mg*

- *Total Carbs 6.8 g*
- *Fiber 1.9 g*
- *Sugar 3.9 g*
- *Protein 1.3 g*

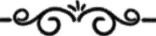

Spinach Soup

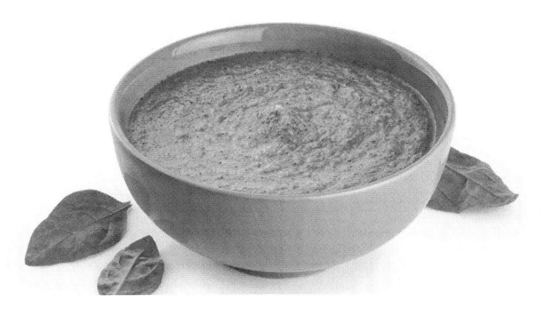

Ingredients
- ➤ 2 tablespoons olive oil
- ➤ 1 large white onion, chopped
- ➤ Pinch of salt
- ➤ 2 large leeks, sliced
- ➤ 2 tablespoons fresh ginger, minced
- ➤ 1 large bunch spinach, chopped
- ➤ 8 cups low-fat chicken broth

> Ground black pepper, as needed

> 1 tablespoon fresh lemon juice

How to Prepare

1. In a soup pan, heat the oil over low heat and cook the onion and salt for about 20 minutes, stirring occasionally.

2. Stir in the leeks and cook for about 10 minutes.

3. Stir in ginger and spinach and cook for about 5 minutes.

4. Add the broth and stir to combine.

5. Now adjust the heat to medium-high and bring to a rolling boil.

6. Now adjust the heat to medium and cook for about 10 minutes.

7. Remove from the heat and set aside to cool slightly.

8. In a blender, add the soup mixture and pulse until smooth.

9. Return the soup to the same pan over medium heat and cook for about 5 minutes.

10. Stir in the lemon juice and black pepper and serve hot.

Preparation time: 10 minutes
Cooking time: 50 minutes
Total time: 1 hour
Servings: 6

Nutritional Values

> *Calories 141*

> *Total Fat 7.1 g*

> *Saturated Fat 1.3 g*

- *Cholesterol 0 mg*
- *Sodium 274 mg*
- *Total Carbs 10.9 g*
- *Fiber 3.2 g*
- *Sugar 2.7 g*
- *Protein 10 g*

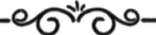

STAGE 4: RECIPES FOR LIFE
BREAKFAST RECIPES

Cheese & Yogurt Bowl

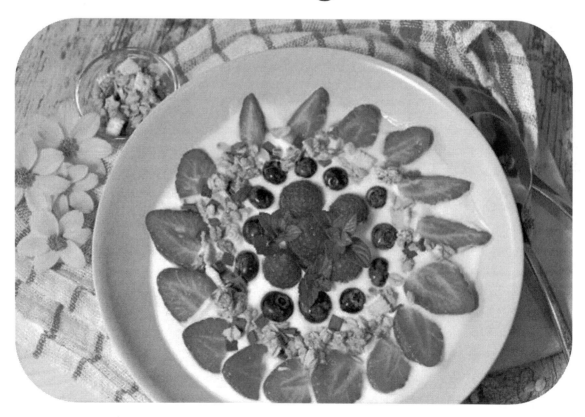

Ingredients

- ½ cup plain fat-free Greek yogurt
- ½ cup low-fat cottage cheese
- 2 teaspoons extra-virgin olive oil
- ¼ teaspoon ground cinnamon
- ¼ cup fresh strawberries, hulled and sliced
- ¼ cup fresh blueberries
- ¼ cup fresh raspberries
- 2 tablespoons walnuts, chopped

How to Prepare

1. In a large bowl, add the yogurt, cheese, oil, and cinnamon, and mix until well combined.
2. Divide the yogurt mixture in 2 serving bowls.
3. Top with berries and walnuts and serve immediately.

Preparation time: 10 minutes

Total time: 10 minutes

Servings: 2

Nutritional Values

- *Calories 204*
- *Total Fat 11.3 g*
- *Saturated Fat 2.2 g*
- *Cholesterol 8 mg*
- *Sodium 270 mg*
- *Total Carbs 12.9 g*

➢ *Fiber 2.5 g*
➢ *Sugar 7.6 g*
➢ *Protein 13.3 g*

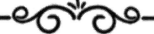

Strawberry Chia Pudding

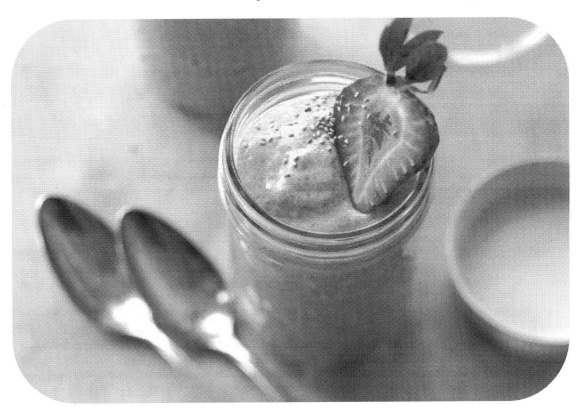

Ingredients
- ➤ 2/3 cup unsweetened almond milk
- ➤ 2 cups frozen strawberries
- ➤ ½ of frozen banana, peeled and sliced

- ➢ 5 large soft dates, pitted and chopped
- ➢ ½ cup chia seeds

How to Prepare

1. Put all ingredients in a high-powered food processor (except for chia seeds) and pulse until smooth.
2. Transfer the mixture in a bowl.
3. Add chia seeds and stir to combine well.
4. Refrigerate for 30 minutes, stirring after every 5 minutes.

Preparation time: 10 minutes

Total time: 10 minutes

Servings: 4

Nutritional Values

- ➢ *Calories 132*
- ➢ *Total Fat 5.7 g*
- ➢ *Saturated Fat 0.5 g*
- ➢ *Cholesterol 0 mg*
- ➢ *Sodium 30 mg*
- ➢ *Total Carbs 24 g*
- ➢ *Fiber 7.9 g*
- ➢ *Sugar 12.8 g*
- ➢ *Protein 3.6 g*

Pumpkin & Cottage Cheese Oatmeal

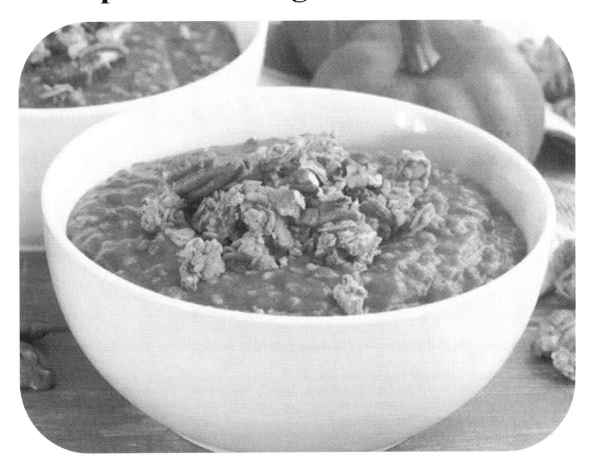

Ingredients

➢ 1/3 cup old-fashioned oats

➢ ½ cup canned sugar-free pumpkin

➢ 1 teaspoon Truvia baking blend

- ➤ 1/8 teaspoon ground cinnamon
- ➤ Pinch of ground cloves
- ➤ Pinch of ground ginger
- ➤ ½ cup no-salt-added 1% cottage cheese
- ➤ 1 tablespoon pecans, chopped

How to Prepare

1. In a microwave-safe bowl, add the oats, pumpkin, Truvia baking blend, and spices, and stir to combine.
2. Microwave on High for about 90 seconds, stirring once after 50 seconds.
3. Remove from the microwave and stir in the cottage cheese.
4. Again, microwave on High for about 60 seconds, stirring once after 30 seconds.
5. Remove the bowl of oat mixture from the microwave and set aside for about 2 minutes before serving.

Preparation time: 10 minutes
Cooking time: 2½ minutes
Total time: 12½ minutes
Servings: 2

Nutritional Values

- ➤ *Calories 206*
- ➤ *Total Fat 5.5 g*
- ➤ *Saturated Fat 1.4 g*
- ➤ *Cholesterol 5 mg*

- Sodium 233 mg
- Total Carbs 27.7 g
- Fiber 4.9 g
- Sugar 3 g
- Protein 12.2 g

Vanilla Crepes

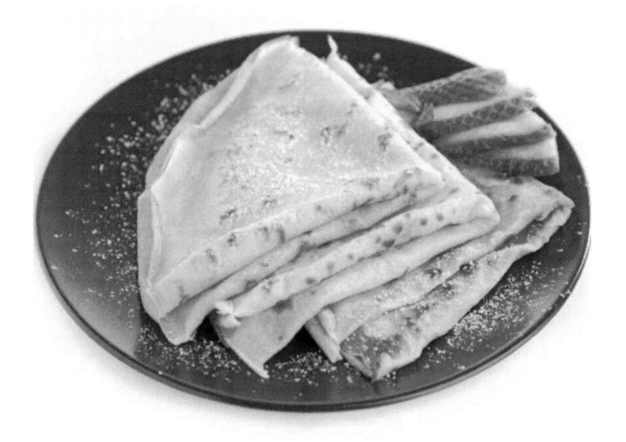

Ingredients

- ➤ 2 tablespoons arrowroot powder
- ➤ 2 tablespoons almond flour
- ➤ ½ teaspoon ground cinnamon

- ➤ 4 eggs
- ➤ 1 teaspoon vanilla extract
- ➤ Olive oil cooking spray

How to Prepare

1. In a bowl, add the arrowroot powder, almond flour, and cinnamon, and mix well.
2. In another bowl, add the eggs and vanilla extract and beat until well combined.
3. Add the egg mixture into the bowl of flour mixture and mix until well combined.
4. Lightly grease a large non-stick sauté pan with cooking spray and heat over medium-high heat.
5. Add the desired amount of mixture and tilt the pan to spread in an even and thin layer.
6. Cook for about 1 minute or until bottom becomes golden-brown.
7. Carefully flip and cook for about 1 minute more or until golden-brown.
8. Repeat with the remaining mixture.
9. Serve warm.

Preparation time: 10 minutes
Cooking time: 18 minutes
Total time: 28 minutes
Servings: 4

Nutritional Values

- ➤ *Calories 107*

- Total Fat 6.3 g
- Saturated Fat 1.5 g
- Cholesterol 164 mg
- Sodium 62 mg
- Total Carbs 5.3 g
- Fiber 0.5 g
- Sugar 0.6 g
- Protein 5.6 g

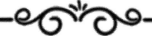

Oatmeal & Cottage Cheese Pancakes

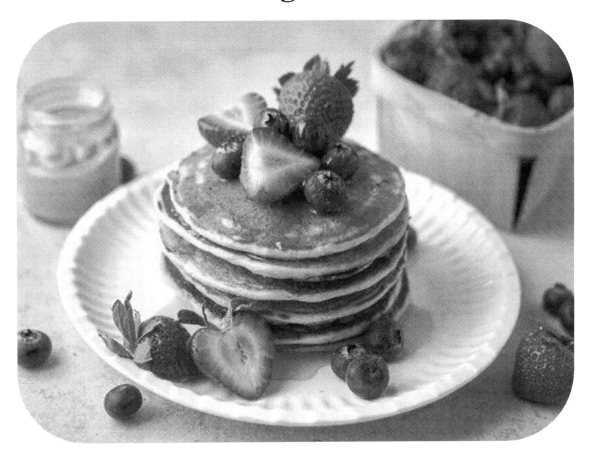

Ingredients

- ➤ ½ cup low-fat cottage cheese
- ➤ ½ cup instant oatmeal
- ➤ 2 tablespoons powdered peanuts

- ➤ 4 large egg whites
- ➤ 1 cup frozen mixed berry blend
- ➤ Olive oil cooking spray

How to Prepare

1. In a blender, add the cottage cheese, oatmeal, powdered peanuts, and egg whites, and pulse until smooth (the mixture should be like a pancake batter).
2. Transfer the mixture into a mixing bowl.
3. Add the mixed berry blend and, with a wooden spoon, gently stir to combine.
4. Lightly grease a large non-stick sauté pan with the cooking spray and heat over medium heat.
5. Add desired amount of the mixture and with a spoon; spread in an even layer.
6. Cook for about 2 minutes or until bottom becomes golden-brown.
7. Carefully flip and cook for about 2 minutes more or until golden-brown.
8. Repeat with the remaining mixture.
9. Serve warm.

Preparation time: 15 minutes
Cooking time: 16 minutes
Total time: 31 minutes
Servings: 4

Nutritional Values

- ➤ *Calories 122*
- ➤ *Total Fat 3.7 g*
- ➤ *Saturated Fat 0.7 g*

- *Cholesterol 2 mg*
- *Sodium 149 mg*
- *Total Carbs 12.7 g*
- *Fiber 2.4 g*
- *Sugar 2.9 g*
- *Protein 10.3 g*

Tofu & Veggies Muffins

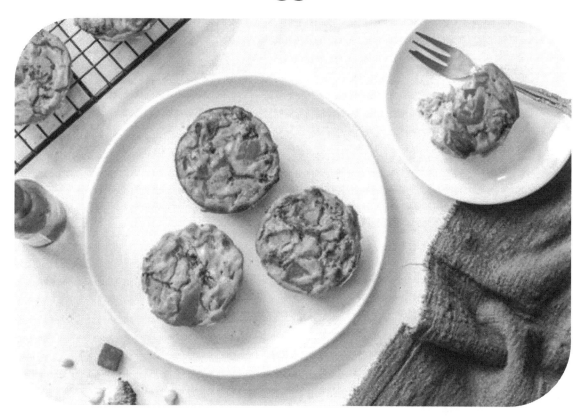

Ingredients

- ➤ 1 teaspoon olive oil
- ➤ 1½ cups fresh shiitake mushrooms, chopped
- ➤ 1 scallion, chopped
- ➤ 1 teaspoon garlic, minced

- ➢ 1 teaspoon fresh rosemary, minced
- ➢ Ground black pepper, as needed
- ➢ 1 (12.3-ounce) package silken tofu, pressed and drained
- ➢ ¼ cup unsweetened almond milk
- ➢ 2 tablespoons low-fat Parmesan cheese, grated
- ➢ 1 tablespoon arrowroot starch
- ➢ ¼ teaspoon extra-virgin olive oil
- ➢ ¼ teaspoon ground turmeric

How to Prepare

1. Preheat your oven to 375°F.
2. Grease 12 cups of a muffin tin.
3. In a non-stick sauté pan, heat the oil over medium heat and sauté the scallion and garlic for about 1 minute.
4. Add the mushrooms and sauté for about 5–7 minutes.
5. Stir in the rosemary and black pepper and remove from the heat
6. Set aside to cool slightly.
7. In a food processor, add the tofu and remaining ingredients and pulse until smooth.
8. Transfer the tofu mixture into a large bowl.
9. Fold in the mushroom mixture.
10. Place the mixture into the prepared muffin cups evenly.
11. Bake for approximately 21–22 minutes or until a wooden skewer inserted in the center comes out clean.
12. Remove the muffin tin from the oven and place onto a wire rack to cool for about 10 minutes.
13. Carefully invert the muffins onto a platter and serve warm.

Preparation time: 20 minutes

Cooking time: 30 minutes

Total time: 50 minutes

Servings: 6

Nutritional Values

- ➤ *Calories 61*
- ➤ *Total Fat 3.1 g*
- ➤ *Saturated Fat 0.6 g*
- ➤ *Cholesterol 1 mg*
- ➤ *Sodium 56 mg*
- ➤ *Total Carbs 3.8 g*
- ➤ *Fiber 0.5 g*
- ➤ *Sugar 1.1 g*
- ➤ *Protein 5 g*

Zucchini Frittata

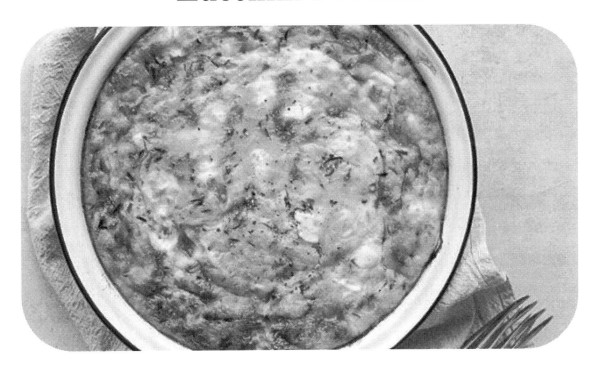

Ingredients

- ➤ 2 tablespoons unsweetened almond milk
- ➤ 8 eggs
- ➤ Ground black pepper, as needed
- ➤ 1 tablespoon olive oil
- ➤ 1 garlic clove, minced

- ➤ 2 medium zucchinis, cut into ¼-inch-thick round slices
- ➤ ½ cup goat cheese, crumbled

How to Prepare

1. Preheat your oven to 350°F.
2. In a bowl, add the almond milk, eggs, and black pepper, and beat well.
3. In an ovenproof sauté pan, heat the oil over medium heat and sauté the garlic for about 1 minute.
4. Stir in the zucchini and cook for about 5 minutes.
5. Add the egg mixture and stir for about 1 minute.
6. Sprinkle the cheese on top evenly.
7. Immediately, transfer the sauté pan into the oven.
8. Bake for approximately 11–12 minutes or until eggs become set.
9. Remove the pan of frittata from oven and set aside to cool for about 5 minutes.
10. Cut into desired-sized wedges and serve.

Preparation time: 10 minutes
Cooking time: 20 minutes
Total time: 30 minutes
Servings: 6

Nutritional Values

- ➤ *Calories 149*
- ➤ *Total Fat 11 g*
- ➤ *Saturated Fat 4.1 g*

- ➢ *Cholesterol 229 mg*
- ➢ *Sodium 232 mg*
- ➢ *Total Carbs 3.4 g*
- ➢ *Fiber 0.8 g*
- ➢ *Sugar 2.1 g*
- ➢ *Protein 10 g*

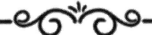

Egg & Black Beans Scramble

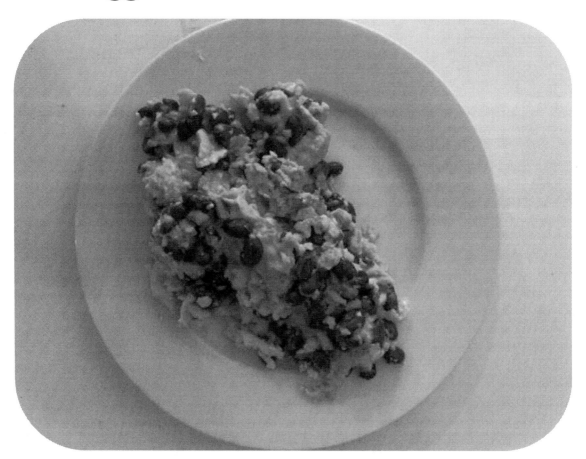

Ingredients

➤ 2 teaspoons olive oil

➤ 5½ ounces canned cannellini beans, rinsed and drained

➤ 1 shallot, sliced thinly

- 2 eggs, lightly beaten
- Ground black pepper, as needed
- 1 tablespoon fresh parsley, chopped

How to Prepare

1. In a non-stick sauté pan, heat the oil over low heat and cook the beans and shallot for about 10 minutes, stirring occasionally.
2. Add the eggs and black pepper and cook for about 3–5 minutes or until done completely, stirring continuously.
3. Remove from the heat and serve immediately with the garnishing of parsley.

Preparation time: 10 minutes
Cooking time: 15 minutes
Total time: 25 minutes
Servings: 2

Nutritional Values

- *Calories 167*
- *Total Fat 9.6 g*
- *Saturated Fat 2 g*
- *Cholesterol 164 mg*
- *Sodium 87 mg*
- *Total Carbs 11.8 g*
- *Fiber 2.9 g*
- *Sugar 0.4 g*
- *Protein 9.3 g*

Sweet Potato & Rosemary Waffles

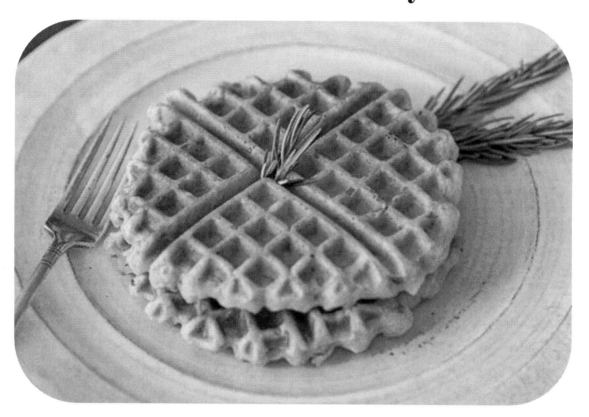

Ingredients

➢ 1 medium sweet potato; peeled, grated, and squeezed

➢ ½ teaspoon dried rosemary, crushed

➢ Pinch of red pepper flakes, crushed

➢ Ground black pepper, as needed

How to Prepare

1. Preheat the waffle iron and then grease it.

2. In a large bowl, add all ingredients and mix until well combined.

3. Place half of the mixture in the preheated waffle iron.

4. Cook for about 8–10 minutes or until waffles become golden-brown.

5. Repeat with the remaining mixture.

6. Serve warm.

Preparation time: 10 minutes

Cooking time: 20 minutes

Total time: 30 minutes

Servings: 2

Nutritional Values

➢ *Calories 65*

➢ *Total Fat 0.2 g*

➢ *Saturated Fat 0 g*

➢ *Cholesterol 0 mg*

➢ *Sodium 25 mg*

➢ *Total Carbs 14.8 g*

➢ *Fiber 2.5 g*

➢ *Sugar 4.6 g*

➢ *Protein 1.4 g*

Eggs with Spinach

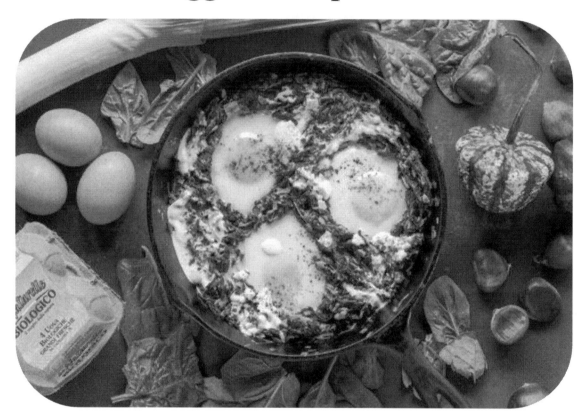

Ingredients

- ➤ 6 cups fresh baby spinach
- ➤ 2–3 tablespoons filtered water
- ➤ 4 eggs
- ➤ Ground black pepper, as needed

- 2–3 tablespoons feta cheese, crumbled
- 2 teaspoons fresh chives, minced

How to Prepare

1. Preheat your oven to 400°F.
2. Lightly, grease 2 small baking dishes.
3. In a non-stick frying pan, put spinach and water over medium heat and cook for about 3–4 minutes, stirring occasionally.
4. Remove from the heat and drain the excess water completely.
5. Divide the spinach into prepared baking dishes evenly.
6. Carefully crack 2 eggs in each baking dish over spinach.
7. Sprinkle with black pepper and top with feta cheese evenly.
8. Arrange the baking dishes onto a large cookie sheet.
9. Bake for approximately 15–18 minutes or until desired doneness of eggs.
10. Remove from the oven and serve hot with the garnishing of chives.

Preparation time: 10 minutes
Cooking time: 22 minutes
Total time: 32 minutes
Servings: 2

Nutritional Values

- *Calories 172*
- *Total Fat 11.2 g*
- *Saturated Fat 4.2 g*
- *Cholesterol 336 mg*

- *Sodium 299 mg*
- *Total Carbs 4.4 g*
- *Fiber 2 g*
- *Sugar 1.5 g*
- *Protein 15 g*

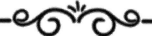

SIDES & SNACKS RECIPES

Broccoli Mash

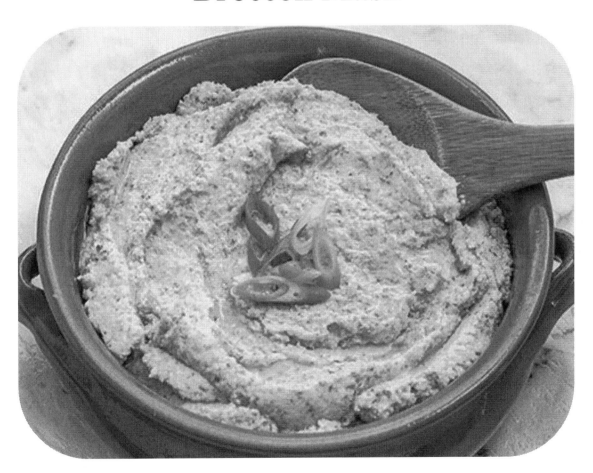

Ingredients

➤ 8 cups broccoli, chopped

➤ ¼ cup olive oil

➤ 4 garlic cloves, chopped

➤ ¼ cup fat-free chicken broth

➤ ¼ teaspoon dry thyme

➤ Salt, as needed

➤ ¼ teaspoon ground white pepper

How to Prepare

1. In a large pan of water, arranger a steamer basket and bring to a boil.

2. Place the broccoli florets into the steamer basket and steam for about 5–6 minutes.

3. Remove the steamer basket and drain the cauliflower completely.

4. Place oil and garlic in a small sauté pan over medium-high heat and cook for about 2–3 minutes, stirring occasionally.

5. Remove the pan of garlic oil from the heat and carefully stir in the broth.

6. Place the cauliflower, garlic mixture, thyme, salt, and white pepper in a food processor, and pulse until fitted with the steel blade attachment. Add the garlic mixture, salt, thyme, and white pepper, and pulse until smooth.

7. Serve immediately.

Preparation time: 10 minutes

Cooking time: 9 minutes

Total time: 19 minutes

Servings: 6

Nutritional Values

➤ *Calories 118*

➤ *Total Fat 8.9 g*

➤ *Saturated Fat 1.2 g*

➤ *Cholesterol 0 mg*

➤ *Sodium 99 mg*

➤ *Total Carbs 8.9 g*

➤ *Fiber 3.2 g*

➤ *Sugar 2.1 g*

➤ *Protein 3.7 g*

Sweet Potato Mash

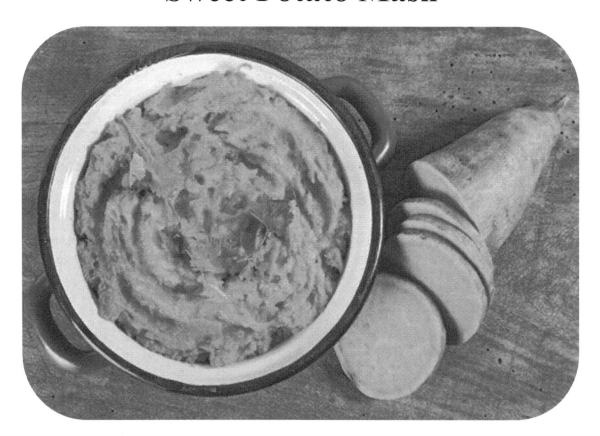

Ingredients

➤ 3 medium sweet potatoes, peeled and cut into chunks

➤ ¼ cup unsweetened almond milk

➤ 1–2 tablespoons maple syrup

- ➢ Salt, as needed
- ➢ ¼ teaspoon ground cinnamon
- ➢ Pinch of ground nutmeg

How to Prepare

1. In a large pan of water, arranger a steamer basket and bring to a boil.
2. Place the sweet potato chunks into the steamer basket and steam, covered for about 15–20 minutes.
3. Remove the steamer basket and drain the sweet potato chunks completely.
4. In a medium-sized bowl, add the steamed sweet potato chunks, and with a potato masher, mash completely.
5. Add the remaining ingredients and stir to combine.
6. Serve immediately.

Preparation time: 15 minutes
Cooking time: 20 minutes
Total time: 35 minutes
Servings: 4

Nutritional Values

- ➢ *Calories 140*
- ➢ *Total Fat 0.4 g*
- ➢ *Saturated Fat 0.1 g*
- ➢ *Cholesterol 0 mg*
- ➢ *Sodium 60 mg*

- *Total Carbs 32.9 g*
- *Fiber 4.5 g*
- *Sugar 3.5 g*
- *Protein 1.7 g*

Lemony Green Beans

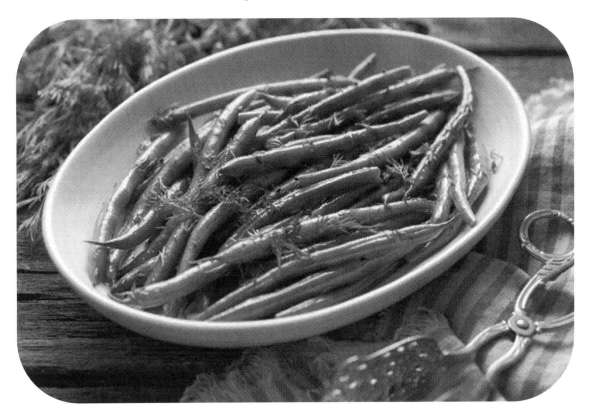

Ingredients

- ➢ 1 pound fresh green beans, trimmed
- ➢ 1 tablespoon fresh lemon juice, plus
- ➢ 1 tablespoon lemon zest, grated
- ➢ 1 tablespoon olive oil
- ➢ Salt and ground black pepper, as needed

How to Prepare

1. In a large saucepan of water, arranger a steamer basket and bring to a boil.
2. Place the green beans into the steamer basket and steam, covered for about 4–5 minutes.
3. Remove the steamer basket and drain the green beans completely.
4. Transfer the green beans into a bowl with the remaining ingredients and toss to coat well.
5. Serve immediately.

Preparation time: 10 minutes
Cooking time: 5 minutes
Total time: 15 minutes
Servings: 4

Nutritional Values

➤ *Calories 67*
➤ *Total Fat 3.7 g*
➤ *Saturated Fat 0.6 g*
➤ *Cholesterol 0 mg*
➤ *Sodium 46 mg*
➤ *Total Carbs 8.5 g*
➤ *Fiber 4 g*
➤ *Sugar 1.8 g*
➤ *Protein 2.1 g*

Roasted Cauliflower

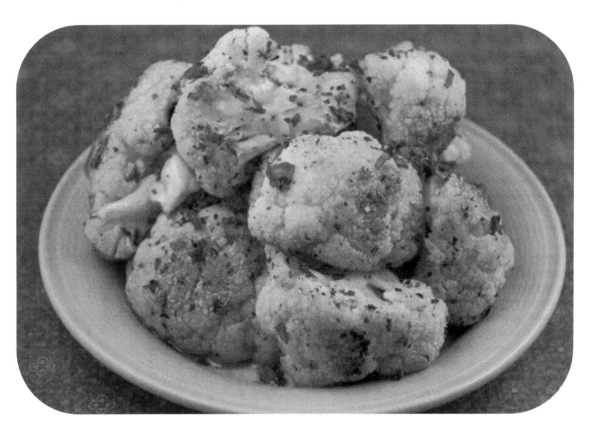

Ingredients

- ➢ 8 cups cauliflower florets
- ➢ ¼ cup extra-virgin olive oil
- ➢ 5 garlic cloves, chopped
- ➢ 2 teaspoons fresh thyme, chopped

- ➤ ¼ teaspoon red pepper flakes, crushed
- ➤ Salt, as needed

How to Prepare

1. Preheat your oven to 450°F.

2. Grease a baking sheet.

3. Place the cauliflower, oil, garlic, thyme, red pepper flakes, and salt, and toss to coat well.

4. Place the cauliflower florets onto the prepared baking sheet and spread in a single layer.

5. Roast for approximately 18–20 minutes or until golden-brown.

6. Serve hot.

Preparation time: 15 minutes
Cooking time: 20 minutes
Total time: 35 minutes
Servings: 6

Nutritional Values

- ➤ *Calories 110*
- ➤ *Total Fat 8.6 g*
- ➤ *Saturated Fat 1.2 g*
- ➤ *Cholesterol 0 mg*
- ➤ *Sodium 68 mg*
- ➤ *Total Carbs 8.2 g*
- ➤ *Fiber 3.5g*
- ➤ *Sugar 3.3 g*
- ➤ *Protein 2.8 g*

Sautéed Spinach

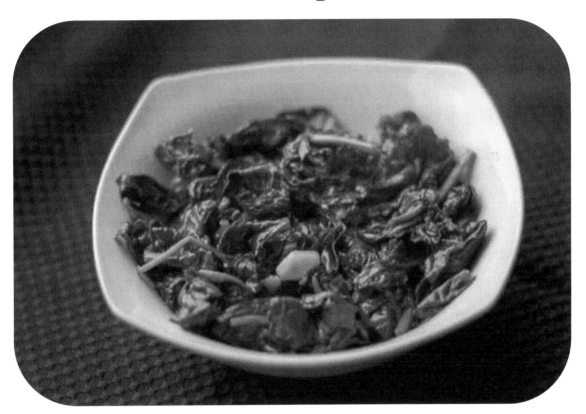

Ingredients

- ➤ 2 tablespoons olive oil
- ➤ 3 garlic cloves, sliced
- ➤ 1 pound fresh spinach
- ➤ Salt, as needed

How to Prepare

1. Heat olive oil in a non-stick sauté pan over medium-high heat and sauté the garlic for about 1 minute.

2. Stir in the spinach and cook, covered for about 2 minutes, flipping the spinach once halfway through.

3. Uncover and drain the spinach completely.

4. Stir in the salt and cook for about 1 minute, stirring continuously.

5. Serve hot.

Preparation time: 10 minutes

Cooking time: 4 minutes

Total time: 14 minutes

Servings: 4

Nutritional Values

➤ *Calories 89*

➤ *Total Fat 7.5 g*

➤ *Saturated Fat 1.1 g*

➤ *Cholesterol 0 mg*

➤ *Sodium 129 mg*

➤ *Total Carbs 4.9 g*

➤ *Fiber 2.5 g*

➤ *Sugar 0.5 g*

➤ *Protein 3.4 g*

Pesto Carrot Sticks

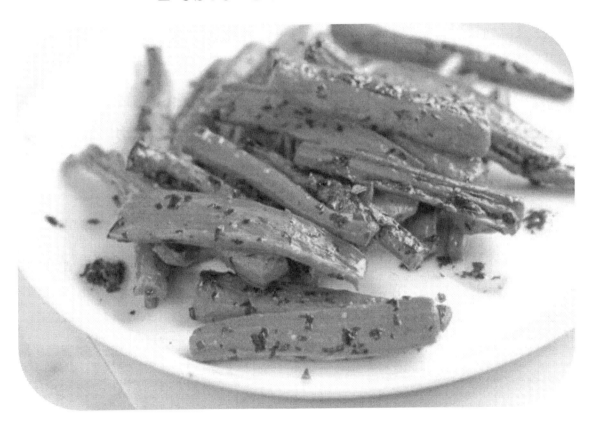

Ingredients

- ➤ 2 carrots, peeled and sliced into 2-inch-long sticks
- ➤ Olive oil cooking spray
- ➤ 2 garlic cloves, chopped
- ➤ ½ of jalapeño pepper, chopped roughly

- ➤ 1 cup fresh basil, chopped
- ➤ 1 tablespoon fresh lime juice
- ➤ 1 teaspoon ground cumin
- ➤ Pinch of sea salt
- ➤ Ground black pepper, as needed
- ➤ ¼ cup olive oil

How to Prepare

1. Preheat your oven to 400°F.
2. Lightly grease 2 large baking sheets.
3. Divide the carrot sticks onto the prepared baking sheets evenly and arrange in a single layer.
4. Spray the carrot sticks with the cooking spray evenly.
5. Roast for about 20 minutes.
6. **For pesto:** In a food processor, add all ingredients (except oil) and pulse until smooth.
7. While the motor is running, slowly add the oil and pulse until smooth.
8. Remove the carrot sticks from oven and toss with pesto.
9. Roast for 5 minutes more.
10. Remove the baking sheet of carrot sticks from the oven and set aside to cool slightly.
11. Serve warm.

Preparation time: 15 minutes
Cooking time: 25 minutes

Total time: 40 minutes

Servings: 4

Nutritional Values

- ➢ *Calories 103*
- ➢ *Total Fat 10.2 g*
- ➢ *Saturated Fat 1.5 g*
- ➢ *Cholesterol 0 mg*
- ➢ *Sodium 68 mg*
- ➢ *Total Carbs 3.7 g*
- ➢ *Fiber 0.9 g*
- ➢ *Sugar 1.5 g*
- ➢ *Protein 0.6 g*

Deviled Eggs

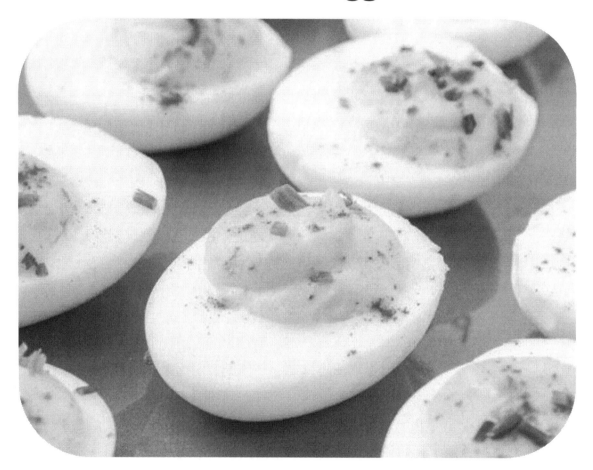

Ingredients

- ➢ 6 large eggs
- ➢ ¼ cup fat-free plain Greek yogurt
- ➢ 2 tablespoons scallions, chopped finely

- ➤ 1 tablespoon fresh chives, minced
- ➤ 1 tablespoon Dijon mustard
- ➤ Cayenne pepper, as needed

How to Prepare

1. In a saucepan of water, add the eggs over high heat and bring to a boil.
2. Cover the saucepan and immediately remove from the heat.
3. Set aside, covered for at least 10–15 minutes.
4. Drain the eggs and let them cool completely.
5. Peel the eggs and, with a sharp knife, slice them in half vertically.
6. Remove the yolks from egg halves.
7. Carefully, scoop out the yolks from each egg half.
8. In a blender, add the egg yolks and yogurt and pulse until smooth.
9. Transfer the yogurt mixture into a bowl.
10. Add the scallion, chives and mustard and stir to combine.
11. Spoon the yogurt mixture in each egg half evenly.
12. Serve with the sprinkling of cayenne pepper.

Preparation time: 15 minutes
Cooking time: 5 minutes
Total time: 20 minutes
Servings: 6

Nutritional Values

- ➤ *Calories 79*
- ➤ *Total Fat 5.1 g*

- ➤ *Saturated Fat 1.6 g*
- ➤ *Cholesterol 186 mg*
- ➤ *Sodium 107 mg*
- ➤ *Total Carbs 1.4 g*
- ➤ *Fiber 0.2 g*
- ➤ *Sugar 0.5 g*
- ➤ *Protein 6.9 g*

Cottage Cheese & Strawberry Bowl

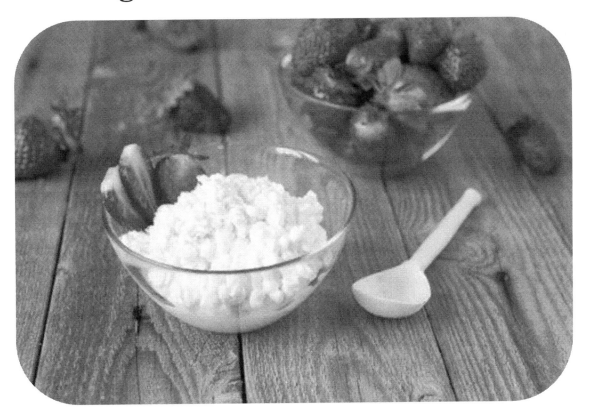

Ingredients
- ➤ 1/3 cup low-fat cottage cheese
- ➤ ¼ cup fresh strawberries, hulled and sliced

How to Prepare

1. In a bowl, add all ingredients and stir to combine.

2. Serve immediately.

Preparation time: 5 minutes

Total time: 5 minutes

Servings: 2

Nutritional Values

- ➢ *Calories 40*
- ➢ *Total Fat 0.8 g*
- ➢ *Saturated Fat 0.5 g*
- ➢ *Cholesterol 3 mg*
- ➢ *Sodium 153 mg*
- ➢ *Total Carbs 2.8 g*
- ➢ *Fiber 0.4 g*
- ➢ *Sugar 1 g*
- ➢ *Protein 5.3 g*

Berries Gazpacho

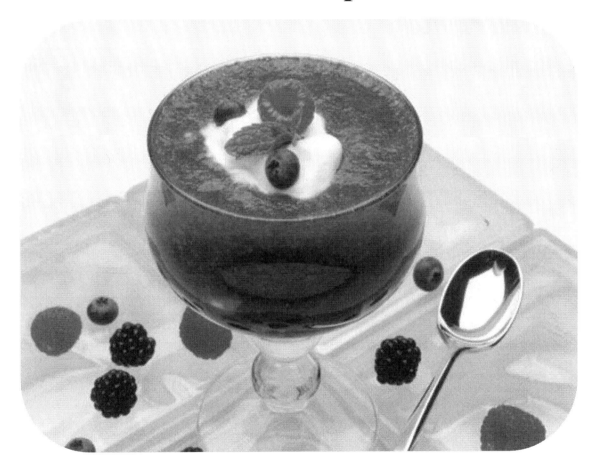

Ingredients

- ➢ 2 cups fresh raspberries
- ➢ 2 cups fresh blueberries
- ➢ 4 cups unsweetened almond milk

➢ ½ teaspoon vanilla extract

How to Prepare

1. In a food processor, put all ingredients and pulse until smooth.
2. Serve immediately.

Preparation time: 10 minutes
Total time: 10 minutes
Servings: 6

Nutritional Values

➢ *Calories 77*
➢ *Total Fat 2.8 g*
➢ *Saturated Fat 0.2 g*
➢ *Cholesterol 0 mg*
➢ *Sodium 121 mg*
➢ *Total Carbs 13.3 g*
➢ *Fiber 4.5 g*
➢ *Sugar 6.7 g*
➢ *Protein 1.5 g*

Black Beans Hummus

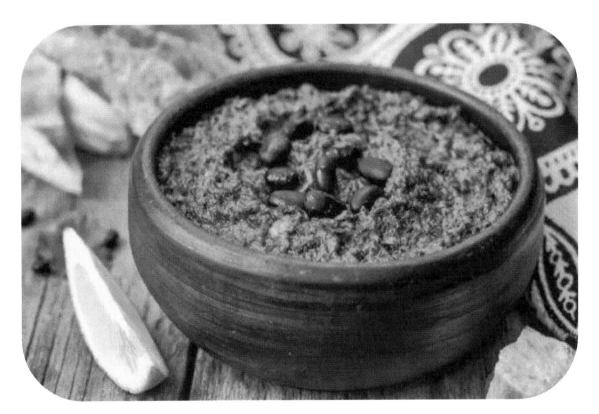

Ingredients
- ➢ 15 ounces canned black beans, rinsed and drained
- ➢ ¼ cup salsa
- ➢ 2 garlic cloves, chopped
- ➢ 3 tablespoons tahini
- ➢ 2 cups boiled cauliflower

- ➢ 1 teaspoon ground cumin
- ➢ 1 teaspoon hot sauce
- ➢ 1 teaspoon extra-virgin olive oil

How to Prepare

1. In a blender, add all ingredients and pulse until smooth.
2. Transfer into a bowl and serve.

Preparation time: 10 minutes
Total time: 10 minutes
Servings: 10

Nutritional Values

- ➢ *Calories 95*
- ➢ *Total Fat 3.2 g*
- ➢ *Saturated Fat 0.5 g*
- ➢ *Cholesterol 0 mg*
- ➢ *Sodium 64 mg*
- ➢ *Total Carbs 12.8 g*
- ➢ *Fiber 4.8 g*
- ➢ *Sugar 0.7 g*
- ➢ *Protein 5.1 g*

VEGETARIAN DINNER RECIPES

Chickpeas Salad

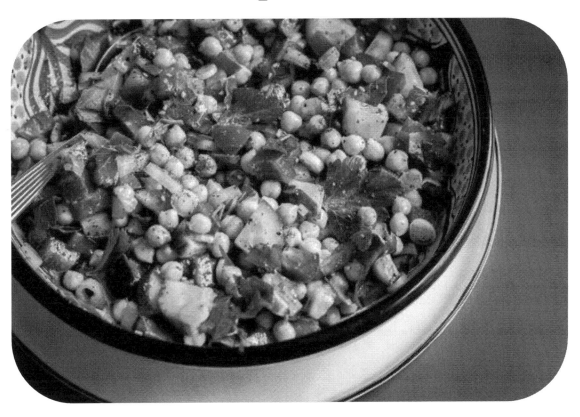

Ingredients

Salad

- 1 (15½-ounce) can chickpeas, drained and rinsed
- 1 head butter lettuce, shredded
- 1 large cucumber, chopped
- 1 red bell pepper, seeded and chopped
- 1 cups tomatoes, chopped
- 1 red onion, chopped
- 2 tablespoons fresh cilantro leaves, chopped
- 2 tablespoons fresh mint leaves, chopped

Dressing

- 1 Serrano pepper, seeded and minced
- 1 garlic clove, minced
- ¼ cup extra-virgin olive oil
- 3 tablespoons red wine vinegar
- 1 tablespoon fresh lemon juice
- ¼ teaspoon red pepper flakes, crushed
- Salt and ground black pepper, as needed

How to Prepare

1. **Salad:** In a salad bowl, add all ingredients and mix.
2. **Dressing:** In another bowl, add all ingredients and beat until well combined.
3. Pour dressing over salad and gently toss to coat well.
4. Serve immediately.

Preparation time: 15 minutes

Total time: 15 minutes

Servings: 4

Nutritional Values

- ➢ Calories 296
- ➢ Total Fat 14.4 g
- ➢ Saturated Fat 2 g
- ➢ Cholesterol 0 mg
- ➢ Sodium 380 mg
- ➢ Total Carbs 37.4 g
- ➢ Fiber 7.6 g
- ➢ Sugar 6.1 g
- ➢ Protein 7.5 g

Quinoa, Avocado & Mango Salad

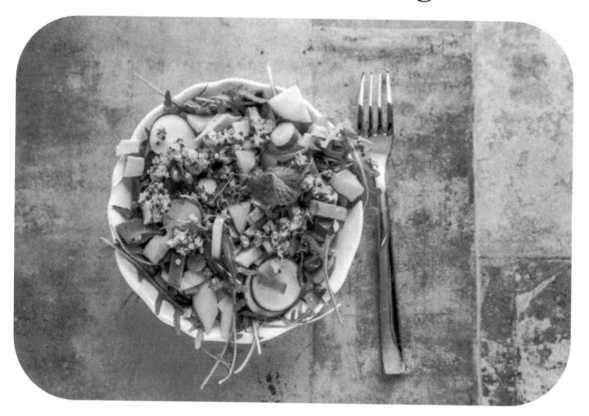

Ingredients

- ➤ 2 cups cooked quinoa
- ➤ 1½ cups fresh mango; peeled, pitted, and chopped
- ➤ 1 avocado; peeled, pitted, and chopped
- ➤ 1 cup radishes, sliced

- ➤ 2 cups fresh baby arugula
- ➤ ¼ cup fresh mint leaves, chopped
- ➤ 2 garlic cloves, minced
- ➤ 2 tablespoons fresh lemon juice
- ➤ 1½ tablespoons olive oil
- ➤ Sea salt, as needed

How to Prepare

1. In a glass salad bowl, put all the ingredients and gently stir to combine.
2. Refrigerate for about 1–2 hours before serving.

Preparation time: 15 minutes
Total time: 15 minutes
Servings: 4

Nutritional Values

- ➤ *Calories 449*
- ➤ *Total Fat 19.2 g*
- ➤ *Saturated Fat 3 g*
- ➤ *Cholesterol 0 mg*
- ➤ *Sodium 78 mg*
- ➤ *Total Carbs 60.5 g*
- ➤ *Fiber 11 g*
- ➤ *Sugar 11.4 g*
- ➤ *Protein 11.5 g*

Sweet Potato & Bell Pepper Soup

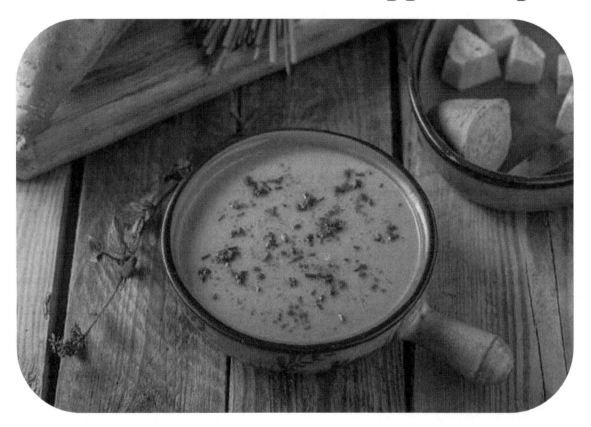

Ingredients

➤ 2 tablespoons olive oil

➤ 1 medium white onion, chopped

➤ 1 red bell pepper, seeded and chopped

➤ 2 garlic cloves, minced

- 1 (1-inch) piece fresh ginger, grated
- 1 teaspoon dried rosemary, crushed
- 1 teaspoon dried thyme, crushed
- 1 teaspoon ground cinnamon
- ½ teaspoon cayenne pepper
- ½ cup tomato puree
- 1 tablespoon maple syrup
- 3 cups low-fat vegetable broth
- 2 large sweet potatoes, peeled and chopped
- 2 tablespoons fresh lemon juice
- Ground black pepper, as needed
- ¼ cup fresh cilantro, chopped

How to Prepare

1. In a soup pan, heat the oil over medium heat and sauté the onion for about 5 minutes.
2. Add the bell pepper, garlic, ginger, dried herbs, cinnamon, and cayenne pepper, and sauté for about 1 minute.
3. Stir in the tomato puree and maple syrup and cook for about 1 minute.
4. Stir in the sweet potatoes and broth and bring to a boil.
5. Simmer for about 10–15 minutes, stirring occasionally.
6. Remove from the heat and set aside to cool slightly.
7. In a blender, add the soup in 2 batches and pulse until smooth.
8. Return the soup in the same pan over medium-low heat and simmer for about 4–5 minutes or until heated completely.

9. Stir in the lemon juice and black pepper and remove from the heat.

10. Serve hot with the garnishing of cilantro.

Preparation time: 15 minutes

Cooking time: 30 minutes

Total time: 45 minutes

Servings: 4

Nutritional Values

- ➢ Calories 219
- ➢ Total Fat 7.6 g
- ➢ Saturated Fat 1.2 g
- ➢ Cholesterol 0 mg
- ➢ Sodium 268 mg
- ➢ Total Carbs 37.7 g
- ➢ Fiber 5.4 g
- ➢ Sugar 8.5 g
- ➢ Protein 2.6 g

Pumpkin & Black Beans Soup

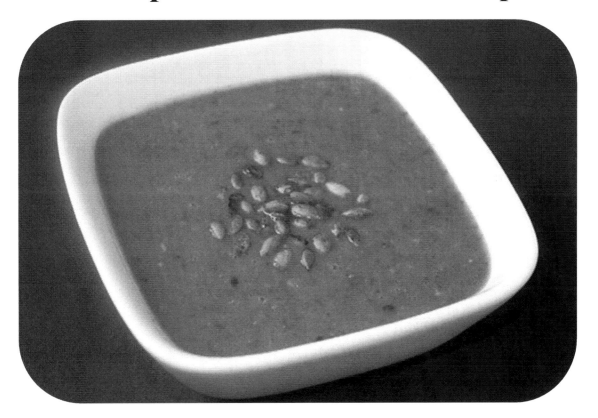

Ingredients

➢ 2 tablespoons olive oil

➢ 1 medium white onion, chopped

➢ 4 garlic cloves, minced

➢ 1 tablespoon ground cumin

➢ 1 teaspoon red chili powder

- ➤ Ground black pepper, as needed
- ➤ 2 (15-ounce) cans black beans, rinsed and drained thoroughly
- ➤ 16 ounces canned sugar-free pumpkin puree
- ➤ 1 cup fresh tomatoes, chopped finely
- ➤ 2 cups low-fat chicken broth
- ➤ ¼ cup fat-free plain Greek yogurt
- ➤ ¼ cup fresh cilantro, chopped

How to Prepare

1. In a soup pan, heat the oil over medium heat and sauté the onion for about 4–5 minutes.
2. Add the garlic, cumin, chili powder, and black pepper, and sauté for about 1 minute.
3. Add the black beans, pumpkin, tomatoes, and broth, and stir to combine.
4. Now adjust the heat to medium-high and bring to a boil.
5. Now adjust the heat to low and simmer, uncovered for about 25 minutes, stirring occasionally.
6. Remove from the heat and stir in yogurt.
7. With an immersion blender, blend the soup until smooth.
8. Serve hot with the garnishing of cilantro.

Preparation time: 15 minutes
Cooking time: 35 minutes
Total time: 50 minutes
Servings: 6

Nutritional Values

- Calories 290
- Total Fat 6.5 g
- Saturated Fat 1.2 g
- Cholesterol 0 mg
- Sodium 65 mg
- Total Carbs 44.7 g
- Fiber 15.6 g
- Sugar 4.1 g
- Protein 16.3 g

Lentils & Quinoa Stew

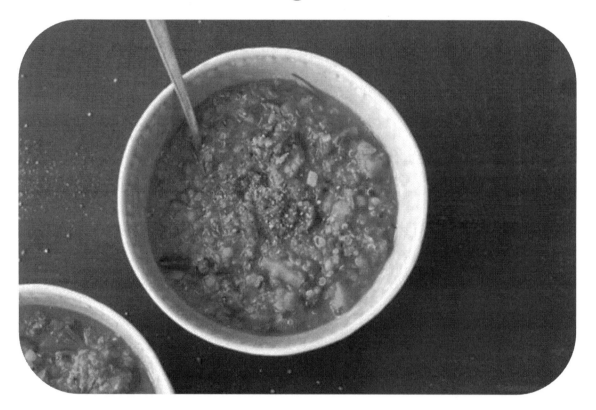

Ingredients

- ➢ 1 tablespoon extra-virgin olive oil
- ➢ 3 carrots, peeled and chopped
- ➢ 3 celery stalks, chopped
- ➢ 1 yellow onion, chopped
- ➢ 4 garlic cloves, minced

- 4 cups fresh tomatoes, chopped
- 1 cup red lentils, rinsed and drained
- ½ cup dried quinoa, rinsed and drained
- 1½ teaspoons ground cumin
- 1 teaspoon red chili powder
- 5 cups low-fat vegetable broth
- 2 cups fresh spinach, chopped

How to Prepare

1. In a heavy-bottomed saucepan, add olive oil and heat over medium heat.
2. Add the celery, onion, and carrot, and cook for about 8 minutes, stirring frequently.
3. Add the garlic and sauté for about 1 minute.
4. Add the remaining ingredients (except spinach) and bring to a boil.
5. Now adjust the heat to low and simmer, covered for about 20 minutes.
6. Stir in spinach and simmer for about 3-4 minutes.
7. Serve hot.

Preparation time: 15 minutes
Cooking time: 33 minutes
Total time: 48 minutes
Servings: 6

Nutritional Values

- *Calories 253*
- *Total Fat 4 g*
- *Saturated Fat 0.5 g*

- ➤ *Cholesterol 0 mg*
- ➤ *Sodium 326 mg*
- ➤ *Total Carbs 43.6 g*
- ➤ *Fiber 13.9 g*
- ➤ *Sugar 7.1 g*
- ➤ *Protein 12.4 g*

Sweet Potato & Kale Stew

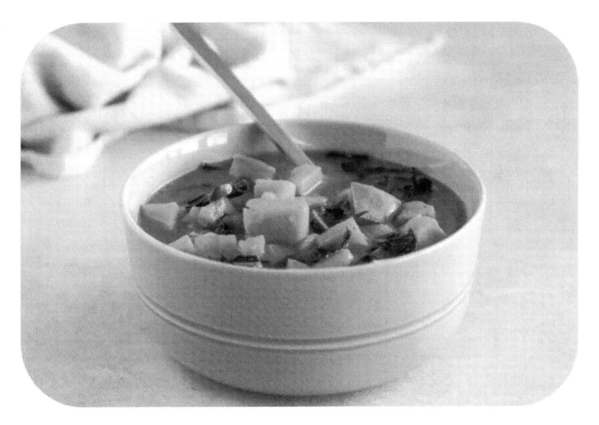

Ingredients

- ➤ 2 tablespoons olive oil

- ➤ 1 medium onion, chopped

- ➤ 1 medium sweet potato, peeled and cut into ½-inch-sized cubes

- ➤ 1 teaspoon fresh ginger, minced

- ➤ 4 garlic cloves, minced

- ➤ 1 Serrano pepper, seeded and chopped
- ➤ ¼ teaspoon red pepper flakes, crushed
- ➤ 1 teaspoon ground cumin
- ➤ ½ cup natural peanut butter
- ➤ 1 (6-ounce) can tomato paste
- ➤ 6 cups low-fat vegetable broth
- ➤ 3 cups fresh kale, tough ribs removed and chopped
- ➤ Salt and ground black pepper, as needed

How to Prepare

1. In a heavy-bottomed saucepan, add olive oil and heat over medium heat.
2. Add onion and sauté for about 4–6 minutes.
3. Add sweet potato and cook for about 5–8 minutes.
4. Add ginger, garlic, serrano pepper, and spices, and sauté for about 1 minute.
5. Add peanut butter and tomato paste and cook for about 2 minutes.
6. Add broth and bring to a boil.
7. Cover and cook for about 5 minutes.
8. Stir in kale, then adjust the heat to low.
9. Simmer for about 15 minutes.
10. Remove the pan of stew from heat and set aside to cool slightly.
11. With a potato masher, blend half of sweet potatoes.
12. Return the pan over medium heat and simmer for about 2–3 minutes.
13. Season with salt and black pepper and serve hot.

Preparation time: 15 minutes
Cooking time: 40 minutes
Total time: 55 minutes
Servings: 6

Nutritional Values

➤ *Calories 280*

➤ *Total Fat 17.2 g*

➤ *Saturated Fat 3.4 g*

➤ *Cholesterol 0 mg*

➤ *Sodium 924 mg*

➤ *Total Carbs 22 g*

➤ *Fiber 4.3 g*

➤ *Sugar 8.7 g*

➤ *Protein 13.4 g*

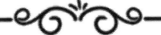

Barley & Lentil Stew

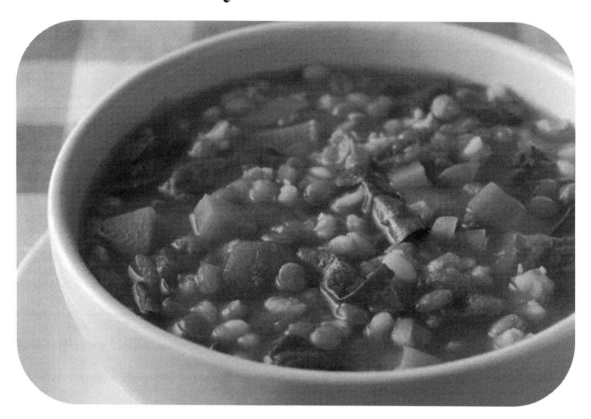

Ingredients

- ➤ 2 tablespoons olive oil
- ➤ 2 carrots, peeled and chopped
- ➤ 1 large onion, chopped
- ➤ 2 celery stalks, chopped

- ➢ 2 garlic cloves, minced
- ➢ 1 teaspoon ground coriander
- ➢ 2 teaspoons ground cumin
- ➢ 1 teaspoon cayenne pepper
- ➢ 1 cup barley
- ➢ 1 cup red lentils
- ➢ 1 (14-ounce) can diced tomatoes with liquid
- ➢ 8 cups low-fat vegetable broth
- ➢ 4 cups fresh spinach, torn
- ➢ Salt and ground black pepper, as needed

How to Prepare

1. In a heavy-bottomed saucepan, heat oil over medium heat and sauté carrots, onion, and celery for about 5 minutes.
2. Add garlic and spices and sauté for about 1 minute.
3. Add barley, lentils, tomatoes, and broth, and bring to a boil.
4. Now adjust the heat to low and simmer, covered for about 40 minutes.
5. Stir in spinach, salt, and black pepper, and simmer for about 3–4 minutes.
6. Serve hot.

Preparation time: 15 minutes
Cooking time: 50 minutes
Total time: 1 hour 5 minutes
Servings: 8

Nutritional Values

- ➤ Calories 265
- ➤ Total Fat 6 g
- ➤ Saturated Fat 1.1 g
- ➤ Cholesterol 0 mg
- ➤ Sodium 817 mg
- ➤ Total Carbs 38.7 g
- ➤ Fiber 13.2 g
- ➤ Sugar 4.4 g
- ➤ Protein 15.3 g

Mushroom & Corn Curry

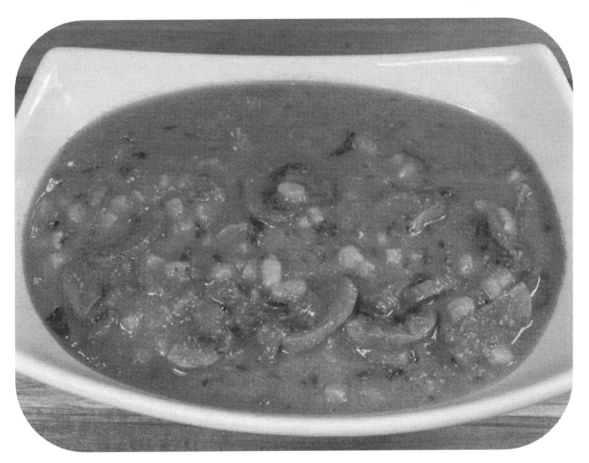

Ingredients
- 2 cups tomatoes, chopped
- 1 green chili, chopped
- 1 teaspoon fresh ginger, chopped

- ¼ cup cashews
- 2 tablespoons olive oil
- ½ teaspoon cumin seeds
- ¼ teaspoon ground coriander
- ¼ teaspoon ground turmeric
- ¼ teaspoon red chili powder
- 1½ cups fresh shiitake mushrooms, sliced
- 1½ cups fresh button mushrooms, sliced
- 1 cup frozen corn kernels
- 1¼ cups water
- ¼ cup unsweetened coconut milk

How to Prepare

1. In a food processor, add tomatoes, green chili, ginger, and cashews, and pulse until a smooth paste forms.
2. In a pan, heat oil over medium heat and sauté cumin seeds for about 1 minute.
3. Add spices and sauté for about 1 minute.
4. Add tomato paste and cook for about 5 minutes.
5. Stir in mushrooms, corn, water, and coconut milk, and cook for about 10–12 minutes, stirring occasionally.
6. Serve hot.

Preparation time: 15 minutes
Cooking time: 20 minutes

Total time: 35 minutes

Servings: 3

Nutritional Values

- ➢ Calories 232
- ➢ Total Fat 15.3 g
- ➢ Saturated Fat 5.1 g
- ➢ Cholesterol 0 mg
- ➢ Sodium 145 mg
- ➢ Total Carbs 24 g
- ➢ Fiber 4.2 g
- ➢ Sugar 7 g
- ➢ Protein 5.3 g

Chickpeas & Pumpkin Curry

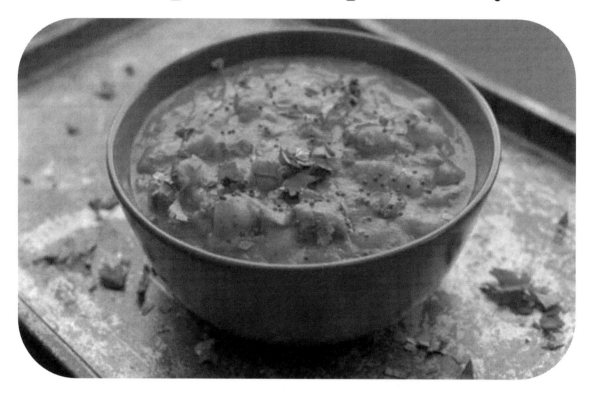

Ingredients

➤ 1 tablespoon olive oil

➤ 1 onion, chopped

➤ 2 garlic cloves, minced

➤ 1 green chili, seeded and chopped finely

➤ 1 teaspoon ground cumin

- ➢ ½ teaspoon ground coriander
- ➢ 1 teaspoon red chili powder
- ➢ 2 cups fresh tomatoes, chopped finely
- ➢ 2 pounds pumpkin, peeled and cubed
- ➢ 2 cups vegetable broth
- ➢ 2 cups canned chickpeas, rinsed and drained
- ➢ Salt and ground black pepper, as needed
- ➢ 2 tablespoons fresh lemon juice
- ➢ 2 tablespoons fresh cilantro leaves, chopped

How to Prepare

1. In a heavy-bottomed saucepan, heat oil over medium-high heat and sauté onion for about 5–7 minutes.
2. Add garlic, green chili, and spices, and sauté for about 1 minute.
3. Add tomatoes and cook for 2–3 minutes, crushing with the back of spoon.
4. Add pumpkin and cook for about 3–4 minutes, stirring occasionally.
5. Add broth and bring to a boil.
6. Now adjust the heat to low and simmer for about 10 minutes.
7. Stir in chickpeas and simmer for about 10 minutes.
8. Stir in salt, black pepper, and lemon juice, and serve hot with the garnishing of cilantro.

Preparation time: 15 minutes
Cooking time: 35 minutes
Total time: 50 minutes
Servings: 4

Nutritional Values

- ➢ Calories 304
- ➢ Total Fat 6.7 g
- ➢ Saturated Fat 1.3 g
- ➢ Cholesterol 0 mg
- ➢ Sodium 805 mg
- ➢ Total Carbs 53.3 g
- ➢ Fiber 13.9 g
- ➢ Sugar 11.6 g
- ➢ Protein 12.3 g

Beans & Sweet Potato Chili

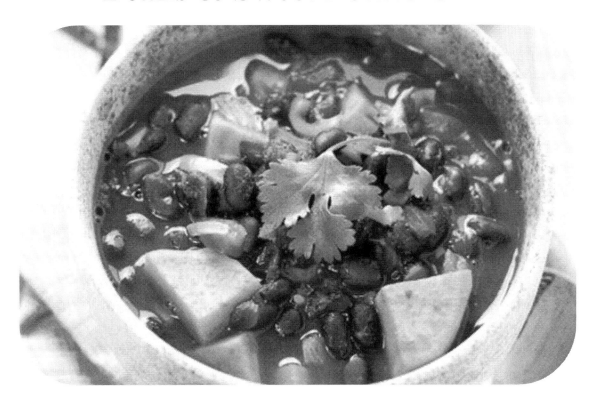

Ingredients

- ➤ 2 tablespoons olive oil
- ➤ 1 onion, chopped
- ➤ 2 small bell peppers, seeds removed and chopped
- ➤ 4 garlic cloves, minced
- ➤ 1 teaspoon ground cumin

- ➢ 1 teaspoon cayenne pepper
- ➢ 1 tablespoon red chili powder
- ➢ 1 medium sweet potato, peeled and chopped
- ➢ 3 cups tomatoes, chopped finely
- ➢ 3 cups canned red kidney beans
- ➢ 1 cup canned corn kernels
- ➢ 2 cups vegetable broth
- ➢ Salt and ground black pepper, as needed

How to Prepare

1. In a Dutch oven, place olive oil and heat over medium-high heat.
2. Add onion and bell peppers and sauté for about 3–4 minutes.
3. Add garlic and spices and sauté for 1 minute.
4. Add sweet potato and cook for about 4–5 minutes.
5. Add remaining all ingredients and bring to a boil.
6. Now adjust the heat to medium-low and simmer, covered for about 1–2 hours.
7. Season with salt and black pepper and serve hot.

Preparation time: 15 minutes

Cooking time: 2¼ hours

Total time: 2½ hours

Servings: 4

Nutritional Values

- ➢ *Calories 373*
- ➢ *Total Fat 9.9 g*
- ➢ *Saturated Fat 1.6 g*

- Cholesterol 0 mg
- Sodium 964 mg
- Total Carbs 59.6 g
- Fiber 16.5 g
- Sugar 15.4 g
- Protein 17.1 g

FISH & SEAFOOD RECIPES

Salmon & Beans Salad

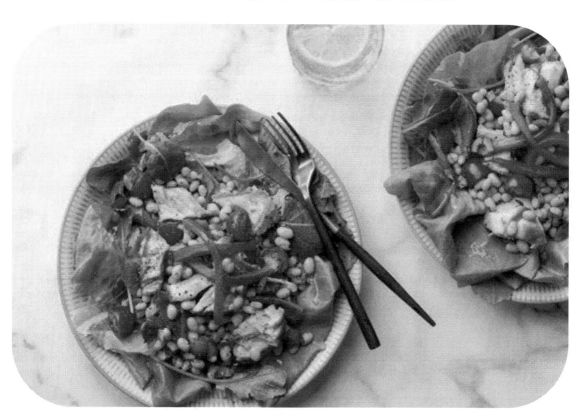

Ingredients

Salmon

➢ 4 (6-ounce) salmon fillets

➢ ½ teaspoon ground cumin

➢ Salt and ground black pepper, as needed

➢ 2 tablespoons olive oil

Salad

➢ 3 cups cooked navy beans

➢ 2 large cucumbers, chopped

➢ 2 tomatoes, chopped

➢ 1 onion, sliced

➢ ¼ cup fresh parsley, minced

➢ 1/3 cup extra-virgin olive oil

➢ ¼ cup fresh lemon juice

➢ Salt and ground black pepper, as needed

How to Prepare

1. Sprinkle the salmon fillets with cumin, salt, and black pepper evenly.

2. In a large non-stick sauté pan, heat the oil over medium heat.

3. Place the salmon fillets in the heated pan, skin-side down and cook for about 3–4 minutes.

4. Carefully flip the side and cook for about 3 minutes.

5. Meanwhile, in a bowl, mix together all salad ingredients.

6. Top with salmon fillets and serve.

Preparation time: 15 minutes

Cooking time: 7 minutes

Total time: 22 minutes

Servings: 6

Nutritional Values

- ➤ *Calories 471*
- ➤ *Total Fat 26.6 g*
- ➤ *Saturated Fat 3.9 g*
- ➤ *Cholesterol 50 mg*
- ➤ *Sodium 301 mg*
- ➤ *Total Carbs 31.1 g*
- ➤ *Fiber 11.1 g*
- ➤ *Sugar 4.1 g*
- ➤ *Protein 30.9 g*

Salmon, Quinoa & Spinach Soup

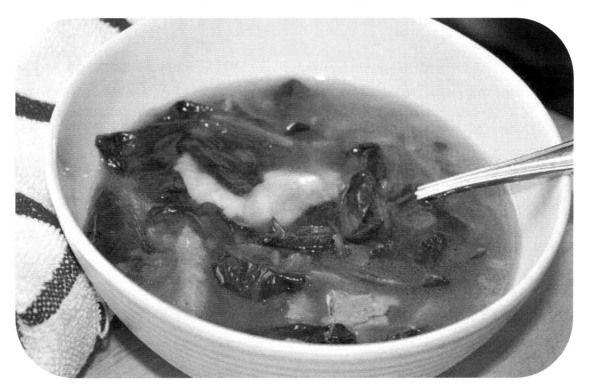

Ingredients

- ➢ 2 cups onions, chopped
- ➢ 1 cup celery stalk, chopped
- ➢ 2 garlic cloves, chopped
- ➢ 2 tablespoons fresh ginger root, chopped finely
- ➢ 1 cup fresh mushrooms, sliced

- ➤ 1 cup quinoa, rinsed
- ➤ 8 cups low-fat vegetable broth
- ➤ 14 ounces salmon fillets
- ➤ 6 cups fresh baby spinach
- ➤ 1 cup fresh cilantro, chopped
- ➤ 1 cup unsweetened coconut milk
- ➤ Salt, as needed

How to Prepare

1. In a soup pan, add onions, celery stalk, garlic, ginger root, mushrooms, quinoa, and broth and bring to a boil.
2. Now adjust the heat to low and simmer, covered for about 45 minutes.
3. Arrange the halibut fillets over the soup mixture.
4. Simmer, covered for about 15 minutes.
5. Stir in remaining ingredients except for scallions and simmer for about 5 minutes.
6. Serve hot.

Preparation time: 15 minutes
Cooking time: 1 hour 10 minutes
Total time: 1 hour 25 minutes
Servings: 8

Nutritional Values
- ➤ *Calories 274*
- ➤ *Total Fat 13.1 g*
- ➤ *Saturated Fat 7.3 g*
- ➤ *Cholesterol 22 mg*

- Sodium 841 mg
- Total Carbs 20.9 g
- Fiber 3.7 g
- Sugar 3.4 g
- Protein 19.6 g

Sweet & Sour Salmon

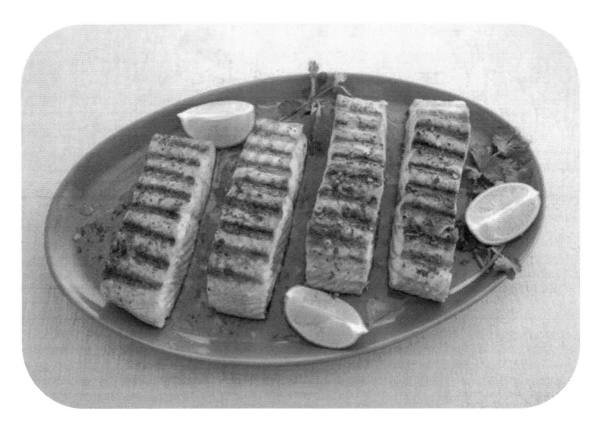

Ingredients

- ➢ 1 scallion, chopped
- ➢ 1 teaspoon garlic powder
- ➢ 1 teaspoon ground ginger
- ➢ ¼ cup organic maple syrup
- ➢ 1/3 cup fresh orange juice

- 1½ pounds salmon fillets

How to Prepare

1. In a Ziplock bag, add all ingredients and seal the bag.
2. Shake the bag to coat the mixture with salmon.
3. Refrigerate for about 30 minutes, flipping occasionally.
4. Preheat the grill to medium heat.
5. Grease the grill grate.
6. Remove the salmon from the bag, reserving the marinade.
7. Place the salmon fillets onto the grill and cook for about 10 minutes.
8. Coat the fillets with reserved marinade and grill for 5 minutes more.

Preparation time: 10 minutes
Cooking time: 15 minutes
Total time: 25 minutes
Servings: 4

Nutritional Values

- *Calories 291*
- *Total Fat 10.6 g*
- *Saturated Fat 1.5 g*
- *Cholesterol 75 mg*
- *Sodium 78 mg*
- *Total Carbs 16.5 g*
- *Fiber 0.3 g*
- *Sugar 13.7 g*
- *Protein 33.4 g*

Salmon with Salsa

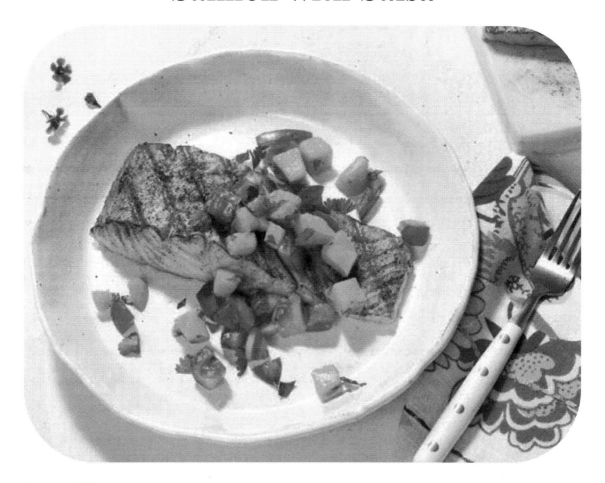

Ingredients

Salsa
- ➤ 2 tablespoons red onion, chopped

- ➤ ½ cup fresh pineapple, chopped
- ➤ ½ cup red bell pepper, seeded and chopped
- ➤ 1 tablespoon fresh lemon juice
- ➤ Ground black pepper, as needed

Salmon

- ➤ 2 (5-ounce) (1-inch-thick) salmon fillets
- ➤ Salt and ground black pepper, as needed
- ➤ 1 tablespoon extra-virgin olive oil
- ➤ 2 tablespoons fresh cilantro leaves, chopped

How to Prepare

1. **For salsa:** In a bowl, add all the ingredients and gently stir to combine.
2. Cover the bowl and refrigerate until serving.
3. Season the salmon fillets with salt and black pepper evenly.
4. In a sauté pan, heat olive oil over medium-high heat.
5. Place the salmon, skin-side up and cook for about 4 minutes.
6. Carefully change the side of fillets and cook for about 4 minutes more.
7. Divide the salmon fillets onto serving plates and serve with the topping of salsa.

Preparation time: 15 minutes
Cooking time: 8 minutes
Total time: 23 minutes
Servings: 2

Nutritional Values

- Calories 284
- Total Fat 16 g
- Saturated Fat 2.3 g
- Cholesterol 63 mg
- Sodium 144 mg
- Total Carbs 8.8 g
- Fiber 1.3 g
- Sugar 6.2 g
- Protein 28.2 g

Salmon in Yogurt Sauce

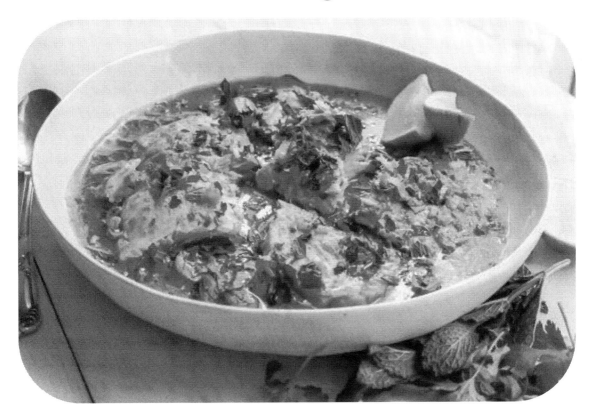

Ingredients

- ➤ 6 (4-ounce) salmon steaks
- ➤ 1½ teaspoons ground turmeric, divided
- ➤ Salt, as needed
- ➤ 3 tablespoons coconut oil, divided

- 1 (1-inch) stick cinnamon, pounded roughly
- 3–4 green cardamom, pounded roughly
- 4–5 whole cloves, pounded roughly
- 2 bay leaves
- 1 onion, chopped finely
- 1 teaspoon garlic paste
- 1½ teaspoons ginger paste
- 3–4 green chilies, halved
- 1 teaspoon red chili powder
- ¾ cup plain fat-free Greek yogurt
- ¾ cup water
- 3 tablespoons fresh cilantro, chopped

How to Prepare

1. In a bowl, season the salmon with ½ teaspoon of the turmeric and salt and set aside.

2. In a large sauté pan, melt coconut oil over medium heat and cook salmon steaks for about 2–3 minutes per side.

3. Transfer the salmon steaks into a bowl.

4. In the same sauté pan, melt the remaining oil over medium heat and sauté cinnamon, green cardamom, whole cloves, and bay leaves for about 1 minute.

5. Add onion and sauté for about 4–5 minutes.

6. Add garlic paste, ginger paste, green chilies, and sauté for about 2 minutes.

7. Now adjust the heat to medium-low.

8. Add remaining turmeric, red chili powder, and salt, and sauté for about 1 minute.

9. Meanwhile, in a bowl, add yogurt and water and beat until smooth.

10. Adjust the heat to low and slowly, add the yogurt mixture, stirring continuously.

11. Simmer, covered for about 15 minutes.

12. Carefully add the salmon fillets and simmer for about 5 minutes.

13. Serve hot with the topping of cilantro.

Preparation time: 15 minutes

Cooking time: 35 minutes

Total time: 50 minutes

Servings: 6

Nutritional Values

➢ *Calories 243*

➢ *Total Fat 14.3 g*

➢ *Saturated Fat 7.2 g*

➢ *Cholesterol 52 mg*

➢ *Sodium 104 mg*

➢ *Total Carbs 5 g*

➢ *Fiber 0.9 g*

➢ *Sugar 3 g*

➢ *Protein 24 g*

Pan-Seared Tilapia

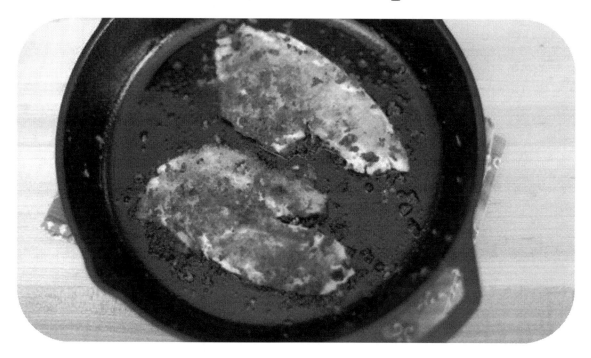

Ingredients

- ➤ 2 tablespoons coconut oil
- ➤ 5 (5-ounce) tilapia fillets
- ➤ 3 garlic cloves, minced
- ➤ 2 tablespoons fresh ginger, grated finely
- ➤ 2 tablespoons unsweetened coconut, shredded
- ➤ 2 tablespoons low-fat chicken broth

How to Prepare

1. In a sauté pan, melt coconut oil over medium heat and cook the tilapia fillets for about 2 minutes.

2. Flip and add garlic, coconut, and ginger, and cook for about 1 minute.

3. Add coconut aminos and cook for about 1 minute.

4. Add scallion and cook for about 1–2 minutes more.

5. Serve immediately.

Preparation time: 10 minutes

Cooking time: 6minutes

Total time: 16 minutes

Servings: 5

Nutritional Values

➢ *Calories 12*
➢ *Total Fat 7.6 g*
➢ *Saturated Fat 5.9 g*
➢ *Cholesterol 69 mg*
➢ *Sodium 55 mg*
➢ *Total Carbs 2.4 g*
➢ *Fiber 0.5 g*
➢ *Sugar 0.2 g*
➢ *Protein 26.9 g*

Haddock in Tomato Sauce

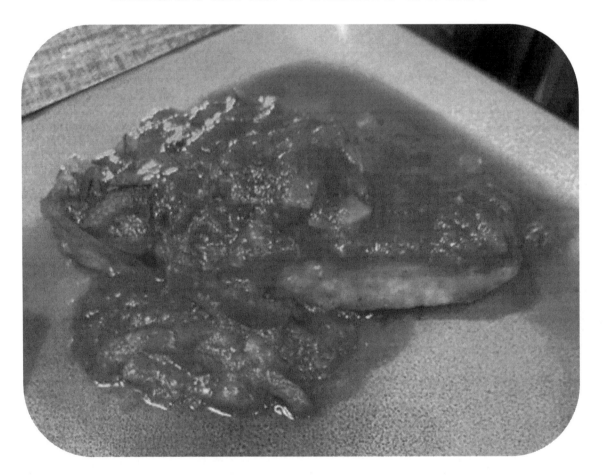

Ingredients

- ➤ 1 tablespoon olive oil

- ➤ 1 cup onion, chopped

- ➤ 2 cups tomatoes, chopped

- ➤ 3 tablespoons fresh cilantro, chopped
- ➤ 1 tablespoon balsamic vinegar
- ➤ 2 (4-ounce) haddock fillets

How to Prepare

1. Preheat your oven to 325ºF.
2. In an ovenproof nonstick sauté pan, heat oil over medium heat and sauté onion for about 4–5 minutes.
3. Add tomatoes and cook for about 2 minutes, stirring continuously.
4. Stir in cilantro and vinegar and cook for about 2–3 minutes.
5. Add haddock fillet and stir to combine with sauce.
6. Transfer the sauté pan into the oven and bake for approximately 12–15 minutes.
7. Serve hot.

Preparation time: 10 minutes
Cooking time: 20 minutes
Total time: 30 minutes
Servings: 2

Nutritional Values

- ➤ *Calories 244*
- ➤ *Total Fat 8.5 g*
- ➤ *Saturated Fat 1.2 g*
- ➤ *Cholesterol 84 mg*
- ➤ *Sodium 111 mg*

- ➢ *Total Carbs 12.5 g*
- ➢ *Fiber 3.4 g*
- ➢ *Sugar 7.2 g*
- ➢ *Protein 29.7 g*

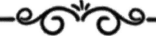

Shrimp Salad

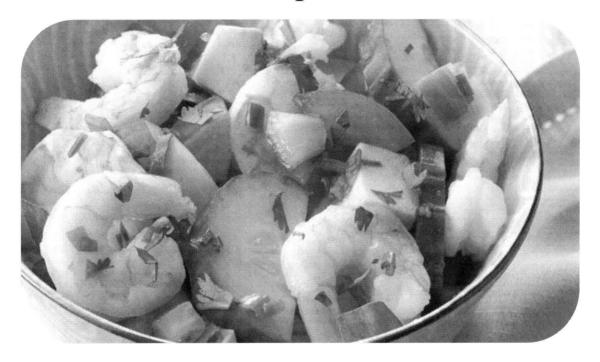

Ingredients

- ➤ 12 medium shrimp
- ➤ 1 large avocado; peeled, pitted, and chopped
- ➤ 1½ cups tomato, chopped
- ➤ 1½ cups cucumber, chopped
- ➤ ½ cup onion, chopped
- ➤ 2 tablespoons balsamic vinegar
- ➤ ¼ cup extra-virgin olive oil

- ➤ 1 teaspoon garlic, minced
- ➤ 2 sprigs fresh cilantro leaves, chopped

How to Prepare

1. In a large pan of the salted boiling water, add the shrimp and lemon and cook for about 3 minutes.
2. Remove from the heat and drain the shrimp well.
3. Set aside to cool.
4. After cooling, peel and devein the shrimps.
5. Transfer the shrimp into a large bowl.
6. Add the remaining ingredients and gently stir to combine.
7. Cover the bowl and refrigerate for about 1 hour before serving.

Preparation time: 15 minutes
Cooking time: 3 minutes
Total time: 18 minutes
Servings: 4

Nutritional Values

- ➤ *Calories 316*
- ➤ *Total Fat 23.7 g*
- ➤ *Saturated Fat 4.2 g*
- ➤ *Cholesterol 139 mg*
- ➤ *Sodium 170 mg*
- ➤ *Total Carbs 11.1 g*
- ➤ *Fiber 4.7 g*
- ➤ *Sugar 3.3 g*
- ➤ *Protein 17 g*

Prawns with Bell Pepper

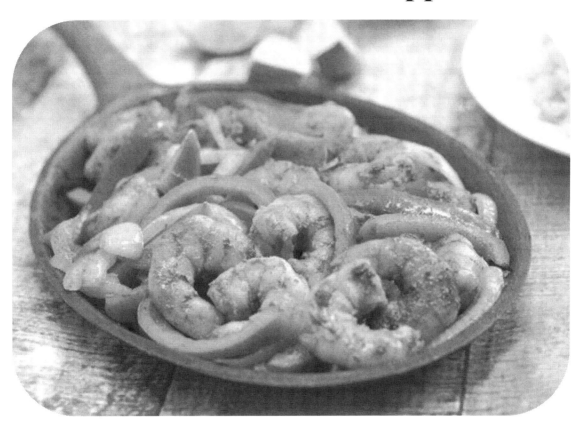

Ingredients

- ➢ 2 tablespoons olive oil
- ➢ 4 garlic cloves, minced
- ➢ 1 fresh red chili, sliced

- 1 pound prawns, peeled and deveined
- 1¼ cups green bell pepper, seeded and julienned
- 1¼ cups red bell pepper, seeded and julienned
- ½ cup white onion, sliced thinly
- ¼ cup low-sodium chicken broth
- Salt and ground black pepper, as needed

How to Prepare

1. In a large non-stick sauté pan, heat olive oil over medium heat and sauté the garlic and red chili for about 2 minutes.
2. Add the prawn, bell peppers, onion, and black pepper, and stir fry for about 5 minutes.
3. Add in the broth and cook for about 1 minute.
4. Serve hot.

Preparation time: 15 minutes
Cooking time: 8 minutes
Total time: 23 minutes
Servings: 4

Nutritional Values

- *Calories 230*
- *Total Fat 9.1 g*
- *Saturated Fat 1.6 g*
- *Cholesterol 239 mg*

- *Sodium 323 mg*
- *Total Carbs 9.7 g*
- *Fiber 1.4 g*
- *Sugar 4.4 g*
- *Protein 27.1 g*

Scallops Salad

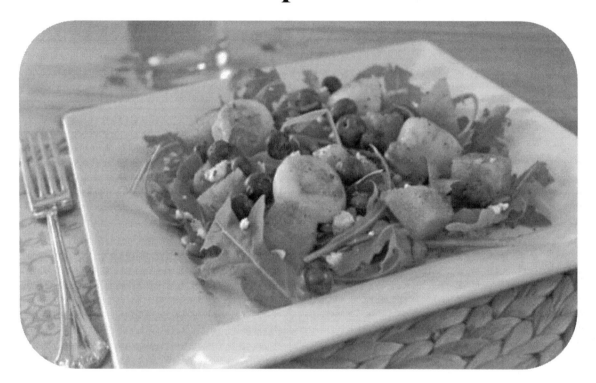

Ingredients

Scallops

- ➤ 1¼ pounds fresh sea scallops, side muscles removed
- ➤ Salt and ground black pepper, as needed
- ➤ 2 tablespoons olive oil
- ➤ 1 garlic clove, minced

Salad

- ➢ 6 cup fresh baby arugula
- ➢ 2 cups seedless watermelon, chopped
- ➢ 1 cup fresh blueberries
- ➢ 2 tablespoons olive oil
- ➢ 2 tablespoons fresh lemon juice
- ➢ Salt and ground black pepper, as needed
- ➢ 2 tablespoons feta cheese, crumbled

How to Prepare

1. Season each scallop with salt and black pepper evenly.
2. In a sauté pan, heat olive oil over medium-high heat and cook the scallops for about 2–3 minutes per side.
3. **For salad:** In a bowl, add all ingredients and toss to coat well.
4. Divide the salad onto serving plates.
5. Top each plate with scallops and serve.

Preparation time: 15 minutes

Cooking time: 6minutes

Total time: 21 minutes

Servings: 4

Nutritional Values

- ➢ *Calories 311*
- ➢ *Total Fat 16.6 g*
- ➢ *Saturated Fat 3 g*
- ➢ *Cholesterol 51 mg*
- ➢ *Sodium 330 mg*

➢ *Total Carbs 16 g*

➢ *Fiber 1.7 g*

➢ *Sugar 9.3 g*

➢ *Protein 26.1 g*

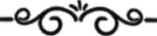

POULTRY DINNER RECIPES

Avocado Strawberry Spinach Salad with Grilled Chicken

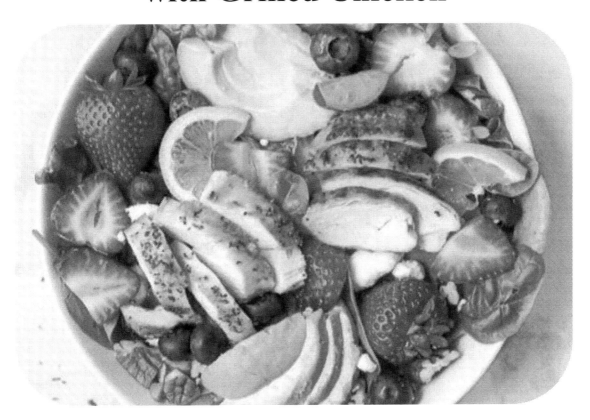

Ingredients

- 2 pounds boneless, skinless chicken breasts
- ½ cup olive oil
- ¼ cup fresh lemon juice
- 1 garlic clove, minced
- Salt and ground black pepper, as needed
- 2 cups fresh strawberries
- 1½ cups fresh blueberries
- 1½ cups fresh raspberries
- 2 large avocados; peeled, pitted, and sliced
- 8 cups fresh spinach, torn
- ½ cup pecans

How to Prepare

1. **For marinade:** In a large bowl, add oil, lemon juice, garlic, salt, and black pepper, and beat until well combined.
2. In a large resealable plastic bag, place the chicken and ¾ cup of marinade.
3. Seal bag and shake to coat well.
4. Refrigerate overnight.
5. Cover the bowl of remaining marinade and refrigerate before serving.
6. Preheat the grill to medium heat. Grease the grill grate.
7. Remove the chicken from plastic bag and discard the marinade.
8. Place the chicken onto grill grate and grill, covered for about 5–8 minutes per side.
9. Remove chicken from grill and cut into bite-sized pieces.
10. In a large bowl, add the chicken pieces, berries, avocado, and spinach, and mix.

11. Place the reserved marinade and toss to coat.

12. Top with pecans and serve immediately.

Preparation time: 15 minutes

Cooking time: 16 minutes

Total time: 31 minutes

Servings: 8

Nutritional Values
- ➢ *Calories 528*
- ➢ *Total Fat 36.9 g*
- ➢ *Saturated Fat 6.8 g*
- ➢ *Cholesterol 101 mg*
- ➢ *Sodium 146 mg*
- ➢ *Total Carbs 16.3 g*
- ➢ *Fiber 7.8 g*
- ➢ *Sugar 6.3 g*
- ➢ *Protein 36.3 g*

Chicken Taco Bowl

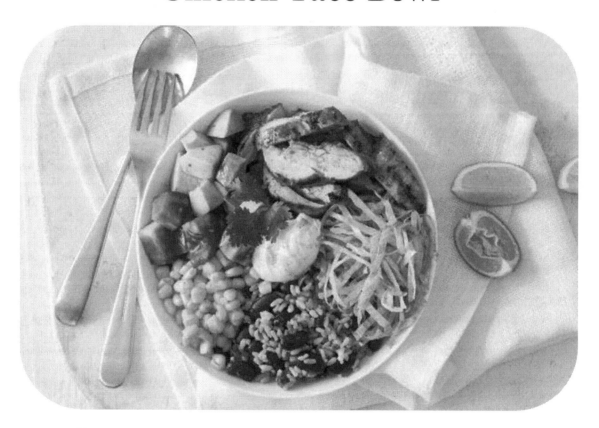

Ingredients

Chicken

- ➤ 4 (4-ounce) boneless, skinless chicken breasts
- ➤ Ground black pepper, as needed

- ➢ 2 tablespoons olive oil
- ➢ ¾ cup low-fat chicken broth

Topping

- ➢ 1 cup cooked black beans
- ➢ 1 cup cooked brown rice
- ➢ 1 cup corn
- ➢ 1 large avocado; peeled, pitted, and sliced
- ➢ 1 large plum tomato, chopped
- ➢ 3 cups lettuce, shredded
- ➢ 2 tablespoons fresh cilantro, chopped

How to Prepare

1. Rub each chicken breast with salt and black pepper evenly.
2. In a sauté pan, heat oil over medium heat and cook the chicken breasts for about 5 minutes.
3. Flip the chicken breast and to with the broth.
4. Cook, covered for about 7–10 minutes or until cooked through.
5. With a slotted spoon, transfer the chicken breast into a bowl and with 2 forks, shred the meat.
6. Add any remaining liquid from the pan into the shredded chicken and stir to combine.
7. Divide the shredded chicken into serving bowls and serve with the topping ingredients.

Preparation time: 15 minutes
Cooking time: 15 minutes

Total time: 30 minutes

Servings: 4

Nutritional Values

➢ *Calories 538*

➢ *Total Fat 26.6 g*

➢ *Saturated Fat 5.6 g*

➢ *Cholesterol 101 mg*

➢ *Sodium 136 mg*

➢ *Total Carbs 35.5 g*

➢ *Fiber 9.3 g*

➢ *Sugar 3.1 g*

➢ *Protein 41.4 g*

Lemony Chicken Breasts

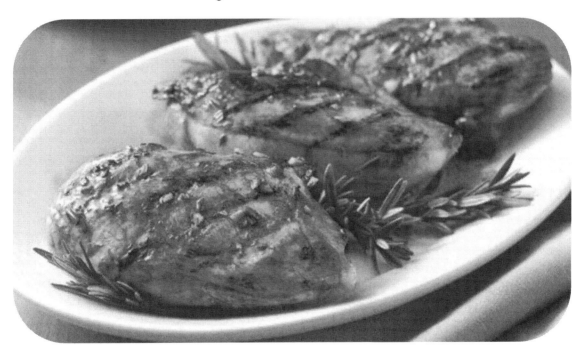

Ingredients

- ➢ 4 (6-ounce) boneless, skinless chicken breast halves
- ➢ ¼ cup balsamic vinegar
- ➢ 2 tablespoons olive oil
- ➢ 1½ teaspoons fresh lemon juice
- ➢ ½ teaspoon lemon-pepper seasoning

How to Prepare

1. With a meat mallet, pound each chicken breast slightly.
2. In a glass baking dish, place the vinegar, oil, lemon juice, and seasoning, and mix well.
3. Add the chicken breasts and coat with the mixture generously.
4. Refrigerate to marinate for about 25–30 minutes.
5. Preheat the grill to medium heat. Grease the grill grate.
6. Arrange the chicken breast halves onto the grill and cover with the lid.
7. Grill for about 12–14 minutes or until desired doneness, flipping once halfway through.
8. Serve hot.

Preparation time: 10 minutes

Cooking time: 14 minutes

Total time: 24 minutes

Servings: 4

Nutritional Values

- ➤ *Calories 258*
- ➤ *Total Fat 11.3 g*
- ➤ *Saturated Fat 1 g*
- ➤ *Cholesterol 109 mg*
- ➤ *Sodium 88 mg*
- ➤ *Total Carbs 0.4 g*
- ➤ *Fiber 0.1 g*
- ➤ *Sugar 0.1 g*
- ➤ *Protein 36.1 g*

Braised Chicken Thighs

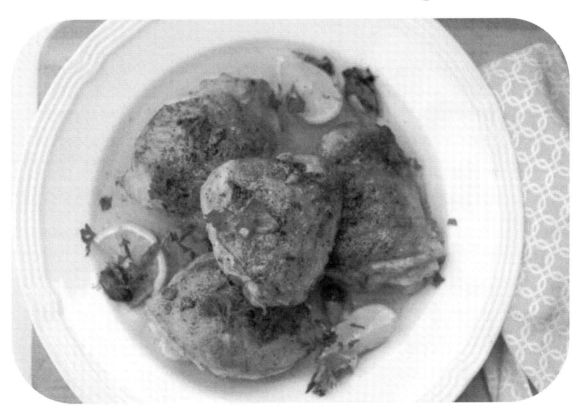

Ingredients

➢ 6 (6-ounce) bone-in chicken thighs

➢ Salt and ground black pepper, as needed

➢ 2 tablespoons olive oil

➢ ½ of onion, sliced

- ➢ 4 cups low-fat chicken broth
- ➢ 2 sprigs fresh dill
- ➢ Pinch of cayenne pepper
- ➢ ½ teaspoon ground turmeric
- ➢ 2 tablespoons fresh lemon juice
- ➢ 2 tablespoons arrowroot starch
- ➢ 1 tablespoon cold water
- ➢ ½ tablespoon fresh dill, chopped

How to Prepare

1. Sprinkle each chicken thigh with salt and black pepper.
2. In a sauté pan, heat oil over high heat.
3. Place the chicken thighs, skin side down and cook for about 3–4 minutes.
4. With a slotted spoon, transfer the chicken thighs onto a plate.
5. In the same sauté pan, add onion over medium heat and sauté for about 4–5 minutes.
6. Return the thighs in sauté pan, skin-side up.
7. Pour in the broth and arrange the dill sprigs over the thighs.
8. Sprinkle with cayenne pepper, turmeric and salt and bring to a boil.
9. Now adjust the heat to medium-low and simmer, covered for about 40–45 minutes, coating the thighs with cooking liquid.
10. Meanwhile, in a small bowl, mix together arrowroot starch and water.
11. Discard the thyme sprigs and transfer the thighs into a bowl.
12. Stir in lemon juice in sauce.
13. Slowly, add arrowroot starch mixture, stirring continuously.

14. Cook for about 3–4 minutes or until desired thickness, stirring occasionally.

15. Add the thighs and stir to combine.

16. Serve hot with the topping of chopped dill.

Preparation time: 15 minutes

Cooking time: 1 hour

Total time: 1¼ hour

Servings: 6

Nutritional Values

➤ *Calories 406*
➤ *Total Fat 18.3 g*
➤ *Saturated Fat 4.5 g*
➤ *Cholesterol 151 mg*
➤ *Sodium 686 mg*
➤ *Total Carbs 4.6 g*
➤ *Fiber 0.5 g*
➤ *Sugar 1 g*
➤ *Protein 52.8 g*

Yogurt & Parmesan Chicken Bake

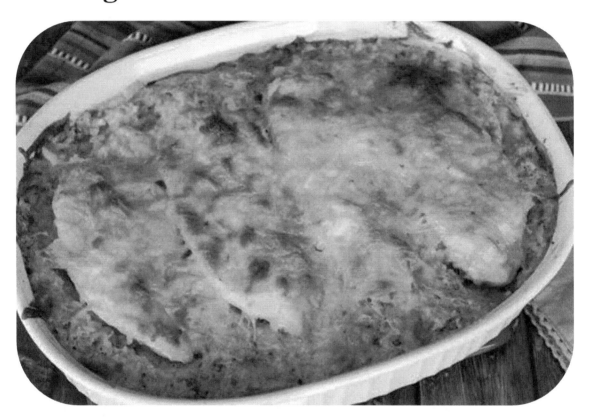

Ingredients

- ➤ 1 cup fat-free plain Greek yogurt
- ➤ ½ cup low-fat Parmesan cheese, grated
- ➤ 1 teaspoon garlic powder
- ➤ Ground black pepper, as needed
- ➤ 4 (4-ounce) boneless, skinless chicken breasts

How to Prepare

1. Preheat your oven to 375°F.
2. Line baking sheet with a greased piece of foil.
3. In a bowl, add the yogurt, cheese, garlic powder, and black pepper, and mix well.
4. Add the chicken breasts and coat with the yogurt mixture evenly.
5. Arrange the chicken breasts onto the prepared baking sheet in a single layer.
6. Bake for approximately 45 minutes.
7. Serve hot.

Preparation time: 15 minutes
Cooking time: 45 minutes
Total time: 1 hour
Servings: 4

Nutritional Values

➢ *Calories 279*
➢ *Total Fat 11 g*
➢ *Saturated Fat 4 g*
➢ *Cholesterol 113 mg*
➢ *Sodium 332 mg*
➢ *Total Carbs 4.9 g*
➢ *Fiber 0.1 g*
➢ *Sugar 0.2 g*
➢ *Protein 37.9 g*

Chicken, Rice & Beans Casserole

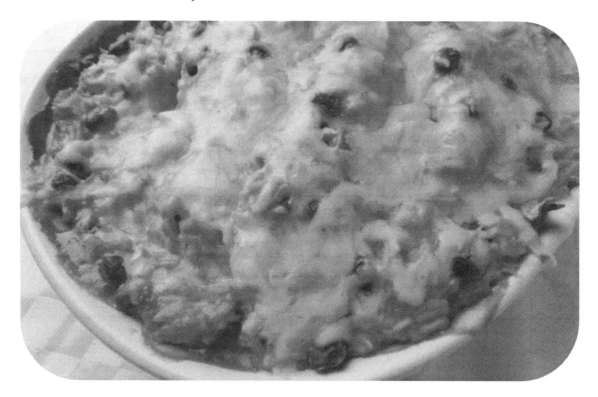

Ingredients

- ➤ 1/3 cup brown rice
- ➤ 1 cup low-fat vegetable broth
- ➤ Olive oil cooking spray
- ➤ 1 tablespoon olive oil
- ➤ 1/3 cup yellow onion, chopped

- 16 ounces cooked chicken breast, cut into small pieces
- 1 medium zucchini, sliced thinly
- ½ cup fresh shiitake mushrooms, sliced
- ½ teaspoon ground cumin
- ¼ teaspoon cayenne pepper
- 1 (15-ounce) can black beans, rinsed and drained
- 1/3 cup carrots, peeled and shredded
- 1 (4-ounce) can diced green chilies
- 2 cups low-fat Swiss cheese, shredded

How to Prepare

1. In a saucepan, add the rice and broth over medium-high heat and bring to a rolling boil.
2. Now adjust the heat to low and simmer, covered for about 45 minutes or until rice is tender.
3. Preheat oven to 350°F.
4. Lightly grease a large casserole dish.
5. Meanwhile, in a sauté pan, heat olive oil over medium heat and sauté the onion for about 4–5 minutes.
6. Stir in the chicken, zucchini, mushrooms, cumin, and cayenne pepper, and cook for about 4–5 minutes.
7. In a bowl, add cooked rice, chicken mixture, black beans, carrots, green chilies, and 1 cup of Swiss cheese and mix well.
8. Transfer the chicken mixture into the prepared casserole dish evenly and sprinkle with the remaining Swiss cheese.

9. With a piece of foil, cover the casserole dish loosely and bake for approximately 30 minutes.

10. Uncover the casserole dish and bake for approximately 10 minutes or until top becomes lightly browned.

11. Remove the casserole dish from oven and set aside for about 5 minutes before serving.

Preparation time: 15 minutes
Cooking time: 1 hour 25 minutes
Total time: 1 hour 40 minutes
Servings: 8

Nutritional Values

➤ *Calories 475*
➤ *Total Fat 12.9 g*
➤ *Saturated Fat 5.9 g*
➤ *Cholesterol 69 mg*
➤ *Sodium 172 mg*
➤ *Total Carbs 54.2 g*
➤ *Fiber 13.1 g*
➤ *Sugar 8.6 g*
➤ *Protein 37.8 g*

Chicken & Veggie Casserole

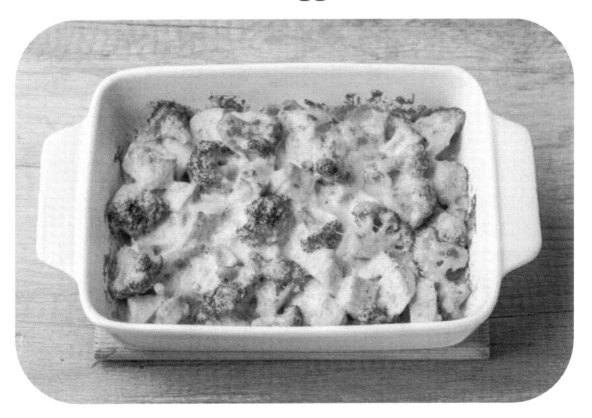

Ingredients

- ➢ 16 ounces broccoli florets
- ➢ ¼ cup water
- ➢ 1 tablespoon olive oil
- ➢ 16 ounces fresh mushrooms, sliced

- ➢ 1 small onion chopped
- ➢ 2 cups boneless skinless chicken breasts, cubed
- ➢ 3 tablespoons almond flour
- ➢ 1½ cups unsweetened almond milk
- ➢ 1 (5.3-ounce) container fat-free plain Greek yogurt
- ➢ ¼ cup low-fat mayonnaise
- ➢ Salt and ground black pepper, as needed
- ➢ ¾ cup Mexican-style cheese blend

How to Prepare

1. Preheat your oven to 350°F.
2. Grease a casserole dish.
3. In a microwave-safe bowl, add broccoli and water and microwave on high for about 3–4 minutes.
4. Remove from the microwave and drain the broccoli completely. Set aside.
5. Heat olive oil in a sauté pan over medium-high heat and cook the mushrooms and onion for about 5–6 minutes, stirring frequently.
6. Add the chicken and cook for about 2–3 minutes.
7. Drain any liquid from the pan.
8. Sprinkle the top of chicken mixture with flour and cook for about 3–4 minutes, stirring continuously.
9. Stir in cooked broccoli and cook for about 1 minute.
10. Add the yogurt, mayonnaise, salt, and black pepper, and gently stir to combine.
11. Remove the pan of chicken mixture from heat and transfer into the prepared casserole dish.

12. With a spoon, spread the chicken mixture evenly and sprinkle with Mexican cheese.

13. Bake for approximately 20 minutes or until cheese is bubbly.

14. Remove the casserole dish from oven and set aside for about 5 minutes before serving.

Preparation time: 15 minutes

Cooking time: 40 minutes

Total time: 55 minutes

Servings: 6

Nutritional Values

➢ *Calories 288*
➢ *Total Fat 16.8 g*
➢ *Saturated Fat 4.5 g*
➢ *Cholesterol 57 mg*
➢ *Sodium 299 mg*
➢ *Total Carbs 13.9 g*
➢ *Fiber 3.6 g*
➢ *Sugar 3.8 g*
➢ *Protein 22.6 g*

Chicken & Sweet Potato Curry

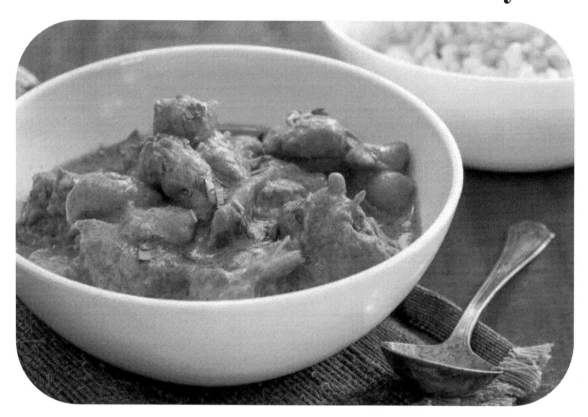

Ingredients

- ➢ 1 pound boneless, skinless chicken breasts, cubed
- ➢ Salt and ground black pepper, as needed
- ➢ 2 tablespoons olive oil, divided
- ➢ ½ of onion, chopped

- 2 garlic cloves, minced
- 1 teaspoon fresh ginger, minced
- 1 teaspoon curry powder
- ½ cup chicken broth
- 2 large sweet potatoes, peeled and cubed
- 1 (14-ounce) can unsweetened coconut milk

How to Prepare

1. Sprinkle the chicken chunks with salt and black pepper.
2. In a large sauté pan, heat 1 tablespoon of oil over medium heat and stir fry the chicken chunks for about 3–4 minutes per side.
3. Transfer the chicken chunks onto a plate.
4. In the same sauté pan, heat the remaining oil over medium heat and sauté onion for about 5–7 minutes.
5. Add garlic, ginger, and curry powder, and sauté for about 1–2 minutes.
6. Add chicken and remaining ingredients and stir to combine well.
7. Cover the pan and simmer for about 15–20 minutes.
8. Stir in salt and black pepper and serve hot.

Preparation time: 15 minutes
Cooking time: 25 minutes
Total time: 30 minutes
Servings: 4

Nutritional Values

- *Calories 325*

- ➢ *Total Fat 13.1 g*
- ➢ *Saturated Fat 4.3 g*
- ➢ *Cholesterol 66 mg*
- ➢ *Sodium 183 mg*
- ➢ *Total Carbs 24.2 g*
- ➢ *Fiber 4 g*
- ➢ *Sugar 1.1 g*
- ➢ *Protein 27.4 g*

Ground Turkey with Veggies

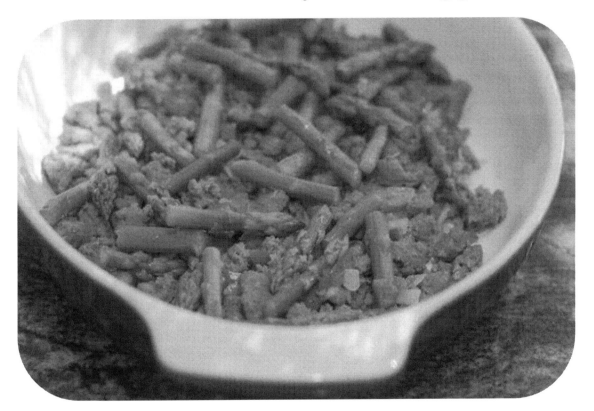

Ingredients

➢ 1¾ pounds lean ground turkey

➢ 2 tablespoons olive oil

➢ 1 medium onion, chopped

➢ 1 cup carrot, peeled and chopped

➢ 6 garlic cloves, minced

- ➢ 2 cups fresh asparagus, ends removed and cut into 1-inch pieces
- ➢ ¼ cup fat-free chicken broth
- ➢ ¼ teaspoon red pepper flakes, crushed
- ➢ Salt and ground black pepper, as needed

How to Prepare

1. Heat a non-stick sauté pan over medium-high heat and cook the turkey for about 6–8 minutes or until browned.
2. With a slotted spoon transfer the turkey in a bowl and discard the grease from sauté pan.
3. In the same sauté pan, heat oil over medium heat and sauté onion, carrot, and garlic for about 5 minutes
4. Add asparagus and cooked turkey and stir to combine.
5. Add in broth, red pepper flakes, salt, and black pepper, and bring to a boil.
6. Now adjust the heat to medium-low and cook for about 6–8 minutes, stirring frequently.
7. Serve hot.

Preparation time: 15 minutes
Cooking time: 25 minutes
Total time: 40 minutes
Servings: 6

Nutritional Values
- ➢ *Calories 328*
- ➢ *Total Fat 19.4 g*
- ➢ *Saturated Fat 3.1 g*
- ➢ *Cholesterol 135 mg*

➢ *Sodium 215 mg*

➢ *Total Carbs 6.3 g*

➢ *Fiber 1.9 g*

➢ *Sugar 2.9 g*

➢ *Protein 37.9 g*

Turkey-Stuffed Zucchini

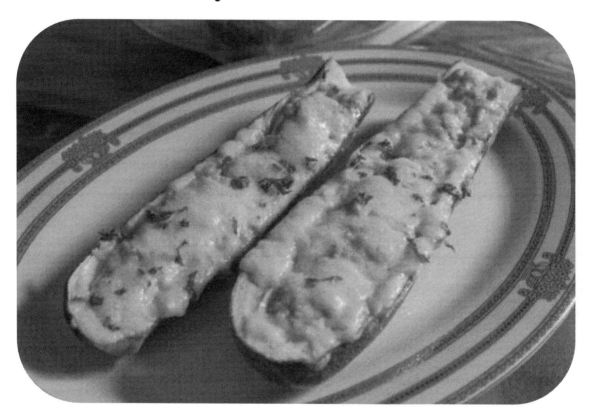

Ingredients

- ➢ 4 medium zucchinis
- ➢ 1 pound lean ground turkey breast
- ➢ ½ cup white onion, chopped
- ➢ ½ pound fresh mushrooms, sliced

- ➤ 1 large tomato, chopped
- ➤ 1 egg, beaten
- ➤ ¾ cup sugar-free spaghetti sauce
- ➤ ¼ cup seasoned whole wheat bread crumbs
- ➤ Ground black pepper, as needed
- ➤ 1 cup low-fat mozzarella cheese, shredded
- ➤ 4 tablespoons fresh parsley, chopped

How to Prepare

1. Preheat your oven to 350°F.
2. Lightly grease a baking dish.
3. Cut each zucchini in half lengthwise.
4. With a knife, cut a thin slice from the bottom of each zucchini to allow zucchini to sit flat.
5. With a small spoon, scoop out the pulp from each zucchini half, leaving ¼-inch shells.
6. Transfer the zucchini pulp into a large bowl and set aside.
7. Arrange the zucchini shells into an ungreased microwave-safe baking dish.
8. Cover the baking dish with a lid and microwave on High for about 3 minutes.
9. Drain the water from the microwave and set aside.
10. Heat a large non-stick sauté pan over medium heat and cook the ground turkey and onion for about 6–8 minutes or until the meat is no longer pink; drain.
11. Remove from the heat.

12. In the zucchini pulp bowl, add the cooked turkey, mushrooms, tomato, egg, spaghetti sauce, black pepper, and ½ cup of the cheese and mix until well combined.

13. Place about ¼ cup of the turkey mixture into each zucchini shell and sprinkle with the remaining cheese.

14. Arrange the zucchini shells into the prepared baking dish.

15. Bake for approximately 20 minutes or until top becomes golden-brown.

16. Serve hot.

Preparation time: 15 minutes
Cooking time: 31 minutes
Total time: 46 minutes
Servings: 8

Nutritional Values:

➢ *Calories 219*
➢ *Total Fat 11 g*
➢ *Saturated Fat 3.2 g*
➢ *Cholesterol 86 mg*
➢ *Sodium 322 mg*
➢ *Total Carbs 11.6 g*
➢ *Fiber 2.7 g*
➢ *Sugar 5.4 g*
➢ *Protein 23.5 g*

PORK & BEEF DINNER RECIPES

Pork & Mango Salad

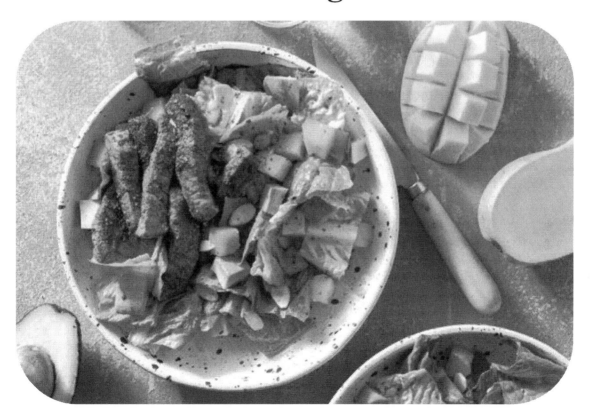

Ingredients
➢ 2 teaspoons fresh rosemary, chopped finely

- ➤ 1 garlic clove, minced
- ➤ 3 tablespoons balsamic vinegar
- ➤ 2 tablespoons extra-virgin olive oil
- ➤ 2 teaspoons fresh lemon juice
- ➤ 1 teaspoon Dijon mustard
- ➤ 1 teaspoon maple syrup
- ➤ ½ teaspoon salt, divided
- ➤ ½ teaspoon freshly ground black pepper, divided
- ➤ 6 cups lettuce, torn
- ➤ 2 cups mango; peeled, pitted and, chopped
- ➤ 1 avocado; peeled, pitted, and chopped

How to Prepare

1. Preheat your oven to 400°F.
2. Grease a large rimmed baking sheet.
3. **For dressing:** In a large bowl, add the rosemary, garlic, vinegar, oil, lemon juice, mustard, maple syrup, ¼ teaspoon of salt, and black pepper, and beat until well combined.
4. Coat the pork tenderloin with 1 tablespoon of the dressing.
5. Reserve the remaining dressing.
6. In the bottom of the prepared baking sheet, arrange the pork tenderloin and sprinkle with the remaining salt and black pepper.
7. Bake for approximately 20–22 minutes.
8. Remove the baking sheet of pork tenderloin from oven and place onto a cutting board for about 5 minutes.
9. With a knife, cut the tenderloin into desired-sized slices.

10. In the bowl of reserved dressing, add the lettuce, mango, and avocado, and toss to coat.

11. Divide the salad onto the serving plates and top with pork slices.

12. Serve immediately.

Preparation time: 15 minutes

Cooking time: 22 minutes

Total time: 37 minutes

Servings: 4

Nutritional Values

➢ *Calories 234*

➢ *Total Fat 17.4 g*

➢ *Saturated Fat 3.2 g*

➢ *Cholesterol 0 mg*

➢ *Sodium 315 mg*

➢ *Total Carbs 21.3 g*

➢ *Fiber 5.6 g*

➢ *Sugar 13.5 g*

➢ *Protein 2.2 g*

Pork with Bell Pepper & Pineapple

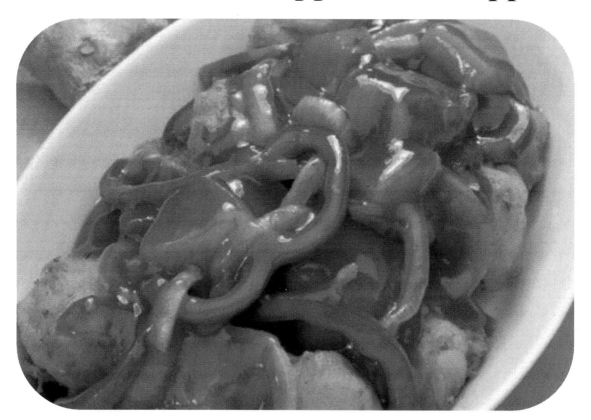

Ingredients

- ➢ 2 tablespoons coconut oil
- ➢ 1½ pounds pork tenderloin, trimmed and cut into bite-sized pieces
- ➢ 1 onion, chopped
- ➢ 2 garlic cloves, minced

- ➢ 1 (1-inch) piece fresh ginger, minced
- ➢ 20 ounces pineapple, cut into chunks
- ➢ 1 large green bell pepper, seeded and sliced
- ➢ ¼ cup fresh pineapple juice
- ➢ 3–4 tablespoons fat-free chicken broth
- ➢ 1 tablespoon fresh lime juice
- ➢ Salt and ground black pepper, as needed

How to Prepare

1. In a large sauté pan, melt coconut oil over high heat and stir-fry pork pieces for about 4–5 minutes.
2. Transfer the pork into a bowl.
3. In the same sauté pan, melt remaining oil over medium heat and sauté onion, garlic and ginger for about 2 minutes.
4. Stir in pineapple and bell pepper and stir fry for about 3 minutes.
5. Stir in pork, pineapple juice, broth, lime juice, salt, and black pepper, and cook for about 3–5 minutes.
6. Serve hot.

Preparation time: 15 minutes
Cooking time: 15 minutes
Total time: 19 minutes
Servings: 5

Nutritional Values
- ➢ *Calories 326*
- ➢ *Total Fat 10.5 g*

- ➤ *Saturated Fat 6.4 g*
- ➤ *Cholesterol 99 mg*
- ➤ *Sodium 141 mg*
- ➤ *Total Carbs 21.1 g*
- ➤ *Fiber 2.5 g*
- ➤ *Sugar 14.6 g*
- ➤ *Protein 37 g*

Peach-Glazed Pork Chops

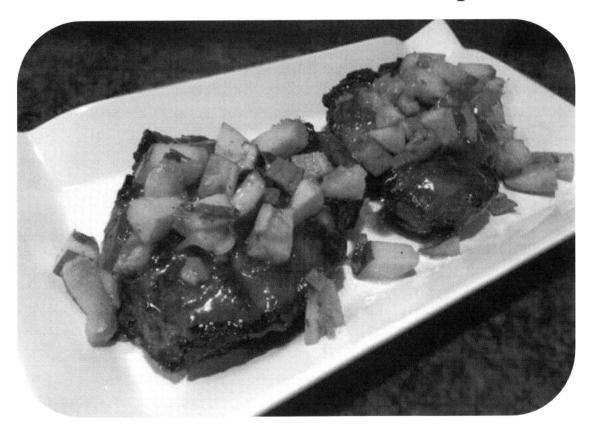

Ingredients

- ➤ 2 boneless pork chops
- ➤ Salt and ground black pepper, as needed
- ➤ 1 ripe yellow peach; peeled, pitted, chopped, and divided
- ➤ 1 tablespoon olive oil

- ➤ 2 tablespoons shallot, minced
- ➤ 2 tablespoons garlic, minced
- ➤ 2 tablespoons fresh ginger, minced
- ➤ 1 tablespoon maple syrup
- ➤ 1 tablespoon balsamic vinegar
- ➤ ¼ teaspoon red pepper flakes, crushed
- ➤ ¼ cup water

How to Prepare

1. Rub each pork chop with salt and black pepper generously.
2. In a blender, add half of peach and pulse until a puree forms.
3. Reserve remaining peach.
4. In a sauté pan, heat oil over medium heat and sauté shallots for about 1–2 minutes.
5. Add garlic and ginger and sauté for about 1 minute.
6. Add remaining ingredients and adjust the heat to medium-low.
7. Simmer for about 4–5 minutes or until a sticky glaze forms.
8. Coat the chops with the remaining glaze.
9. Heat a nonstick sauté pan over medium-high heat and sear the chops for about 4 minutes per side.
10. Transfer the chops onto a plate and coat with the remaining glaze evenly.
11. Top with reserved chopped peach and serve.

Preparation time: 15 minutes
Cooking time: 16 minutes

Total time: 31 minutes

Servings: 2

Nutritional Values

➤ *Calories 610*

➤ *Total Fat 42.9 g*

➤ *Saturated Fat 14.3 g*

➤ *Cholesterol 122 mg*

➤ *Sodium 183 mg*

➤ *Total Carbs 22.2 g*

➤ *Fiber 2.1 g*

➤ *Sugar 13.3 g*

➤ *Protein 33.9 g*

Pork & Beans Stew

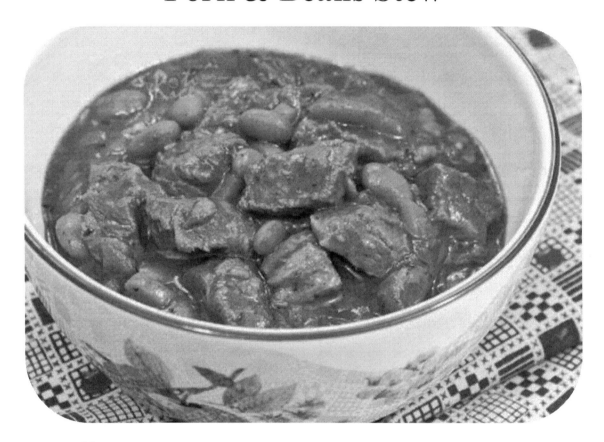

Ingredients
➢ 1 pound dried Great Northern beans

➢ 3½ cups low-fat chicken broth

➢ 1 onion, chopped

➢ 1 (14-ounce) can crushed tomatoes

- ➤ 3 carrots, peeled and cut into ½-inch pieces
- ➤ 2 pounds pork shoulder, cut into 1-inch chunks
- ➤ 2 tablespoons fresh parsley
- ➤ 2 tablespoons fresh thyme
- ➤ 1 teaspoon ground allspice
- ➤ Salt and ground black pepper, as needed

How to Prepare

1. Preheat your oven to 250°F.

2. In a saucepan of water, add the beans and cook for about 20 minutes.

3. Remove the saucepan from heat and then drain the beans.

4. In a large casserole dish, place the beans and remaining ingredients (except for wine) and stir to combine.

5. Cover the casserole dish and bake for approximately 3 hours.

6. Serve hot.

Preparation time: 15 minutes

Cooking time: 3 hours 20 minutes

Total time: 3 hours 35 minutes

Servings: 6

Nutritional Values

- ➤ *Calories 659*
- ➤ *Total Fat 33.3 g*
- ➤ *Saturated Fat 12.2 g*
- ➤ *Cholesterol 136 mg*
- ➤ *Sodium 398 mg*
- ➤ *Total Carbs 57.1 g*

- ➤ *Fiber 31 g*
- ➤ *Sugar 8.1 g*
- ➤ *Protein 57.1 g*

Pork Chops in Sauce

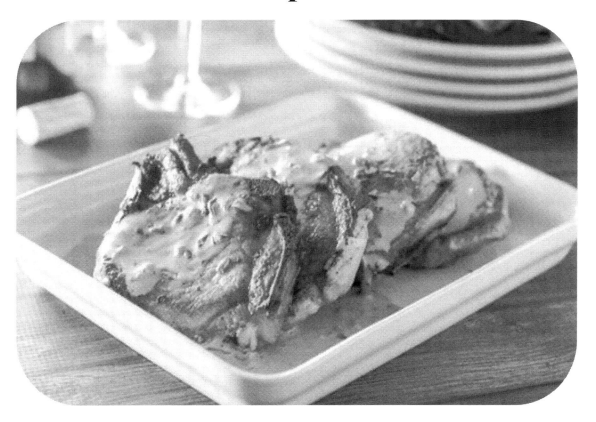

Ingredients

- ➢ 2 garlic cloves, chopped
- ➢ 1 small jalapeño pepper, chopped
- ➢ ¼ cup fresh cilantro leaves
- ➢ 1½ teaspoons ground turmeric, divided

- ➤ 2 tablespoons fresh lime juice
- ➤ 1 (13½-ounce) can unsweetened coconut milk
- ➤ 4 (½-inch thick) pork chops
- ➤ Salt, as needed
- ➤ 1 tablespoon coconut oil
- ➤ 1 shallot, chopped finely

How to Prepare

1. In a blender, add garlic, jalapeño pepper, cilantro, 1 teaspoon of ground turmeric, lime juice, and coconut milk, and pulse until smooth.
2. Sprinkle the pork with salt and remaining turmeric evenly.
3. In a sauté pan, melt coconut oil over medium-high heat and sauté shallots for about 1 minute.
4. Add chops and cook for about 2 minutes per side.
5. Transfer the chops into a bowl.
6. Add coconut milk mixture and bring to a boil.
7. Now adjust the heat to medium and simmer, stirring occasionally for about 5 minutes.
8. Stir in pork chops and cook for about 3–5 minutes.
9. Serve hot.

Preparation time: 15 minutes
Cooking time: 15 minutes
Total time: 30 minutes
Servings: 4

Nutritional Values

➤ Calories 511

➤ Total Fat 40.3 g

➤ Saturated Fat 17. g

➤ Cholesterol 122 mg

➤ Sodium 140 mg

➤ Total Carbs 3 g

➤ Fiber 0.7 g

➤ Sugar 0.2 g

➤ Protein 32.2 g

Steak & Peach Salad

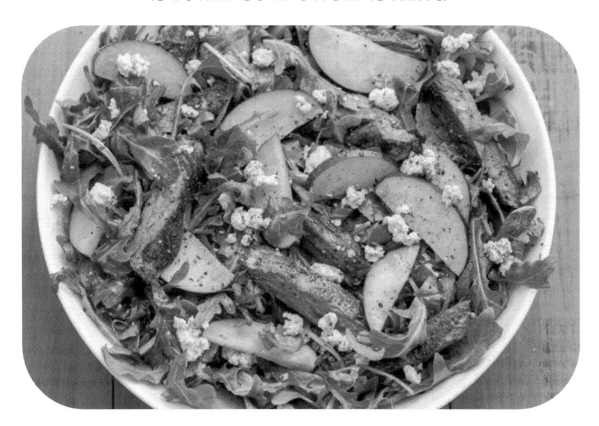

Ingredients

- ➤ 4 teaspoons fresh lemon juice, divided
- ➤ 1½ tablespoons extra-virgin olive oil, divided
- ➤ Salt and ground black pepper, as needed
- ➤ 1 pound flank steak, trimmed

- ➤ Olive oil cooking spray
- ➤ 1 teaspoon maple syrup
- ➤ 8 cups fresh baby arugula
- ➤ 3 plums, pitted and sliced thinly
- ➤ ¼ cup feta cheese, crumbled

How to Prepare

1. In a bowl, put 1 teaspoon of lemon juice, 1½ teaspoons of extra-virgin olive oil, salt, and black pepper, and mix well.
2. Add the steak and coat with mixture generously.
3. Grease a non-stick sauté pan with a little cooking spray and heat over medium-high heat.
4. Add the steak and cook for about 5–6 minutes per side.
5. Transfer the steak onto a cutting board and set aside for about 10 minutes before slicing.
6. With a sharp knife, cut the beef steak diagonally across the grain in desired-sized slices.
7. In a large bowl, add the remaining lemon juice, oil, maple syrup, sea salt, and black pepper, and beat until well combined.
8. Add the arugula and toss to coat well.
9. Divide the arugula onto 4 serving plates.
10. Top with beef slices, peach slices, and cheese evenly and serve.

Preparation time: 15 minutes
Cooking time: 12 minutes

Total time: 27 minutes

Servings: 4

Nutritional Values

- ➤ *Calories 328*
- ➤ *Total Fat 17.1 g*
- ➤ *Saturated Fat 6.1 g*
- ➤ *Cholesterol 71 mg*
- ➤ *Sodium 219 mg*
- ➤ *Total Carbs 9.1 g*
- ➤ *Fiber 1.3 g*
- ➤ *Sugar 7.6 g*
- ➤ *Protein 34.3 g*

Steak with Salsa

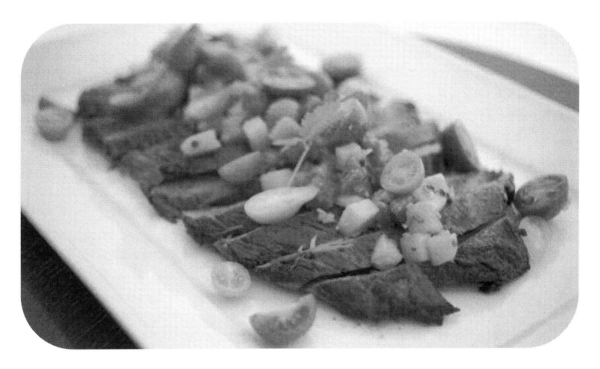

Ingredients

Steak

- ➤ 2 garlic cloves, minced
- ➤ ½ teaspoon ground cumin
- ➤ ¼ teaspoon ground coriander
- ➤ ¼ teaspoon cayenne pepper
- ➤ Pinch of sea salt

- ➤ Ground black pepper, as needed
- ➤ 2 tablespoons fresh lemon juice
- ➤ 1 (1-pound) flank steak, trimmed
- ➤ Olive oil cooking spray

Salsa

- ➤ 1 cup mango; peeled, pitted, and cubed
- ➤ ½ cup yellow grape tomatoes, quartered
- ➤ ½ cup red grape tomatoes, quartered
- ➤ ¼ cup red onion, chopped
- ➤ 2 tablespoons fresh cilantro
- ➤ 1 tablespoon fresh lemon juice
- ➤ Pinch of sea salt
- ➤ Ground black pepper, as needed

How to Prepare

1. **For steak:** In a large bowl, add all the garlic, spices, salt, black pepper, and lemon juice, and mix until well combined.
2. Add the steak and coat with the spice mixture generously.
3. Set aside at room temperature for about 25–30 minutes.
4. Preheat the grill to medium-high heat. Grease the grill grate with cooking spray.
5. Place the flank steak onto the grill and cook for about 6 minutes per side.
6. Remove the steak from the grill and place onto a cutting board for about 10 minutes before slicing.
7. **For salsa:** In a bowl, add all the ingredients and gently stir to combine.

8. With a knife, cut the steak into desired-sized slices.

9. Divide the steak slices onto serving plates and serve with the topping of salsa.

Preparation time: 15 minutes

Cooking time: 12 minutes

Total time: 27 minutes

Servings: 4

Nutritional Values

➤ *Calories 262*
➤ *Total Fat 9.9 g*
➤ *Saturated Fat 4.1 g*
➤ *Cholesterol 62 mg*
➤ *Sodium 128 mg*
➤ *Total Carbs 9.5 g*
➤ *Fiber 1.5 g*
➤ *Sugar 7.4 g*
➤ *Protein 32.6 g*

Beef with Cauliflower

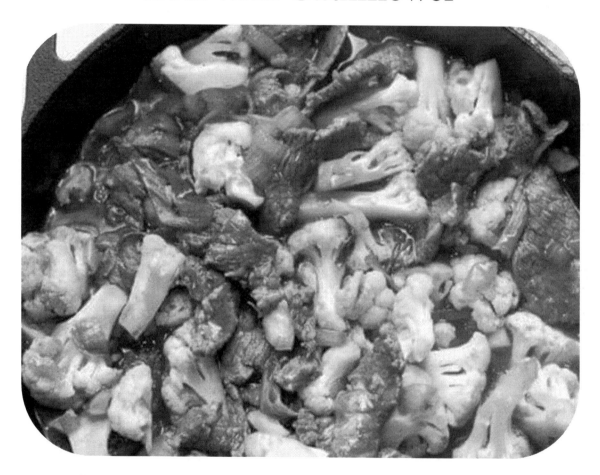

Ingredients
- ➤ 1 tablespoon olive oil
- ➤ 4 garlic cloves, minced
- ➤ 1 pound beef sirloin steak, cut into bite-sized pieces

- ➤ 3½ cups cauliflower florets
- ➤ 3 tablespoons low-fat chicken broth
- ➤ Salt and ground black pepper, as needed
- ➤ 2 tablespoons fresh cilantro leaves, chopped

How to Prepare

1. In a sauté pan, heat olive oil over medium heat and sauté the garlic for about 1 minute.
2. Add the beef pieces and stir to combine.
3. Now adjust the heat to medium-high and cook for about 6–8 minutes or until browned from all sides.
4. Meanwhile, in a pan of boiling water, add the cauliflower and cook for about 5–6 minutes.
5. Remove from the heat and drain the cauliflower completely.
6. Add the cauliflower and broth in sauté pan with beef and cook for about 2–3 minutes.
7. Stir in the black pepper and remove from the heat.
8. Serve hot with the garnishing of cilantro.

Preparation time: 15 minutes
Cooking time: 12 minutes
Total time: 27 minutes
Servings: 4

Nutritional Values

- ➤ *Calories 269*

- ➤ *Total Fat 10.8 g*
- ➤ *Saturated Fat 3.2 g*
- ➤ *Cholesterol 101 mg*
- ➤ *Sodium 147 mg*
- ➤ *Total Carbs 5.7 g*
- ➤ *Fiber 2.3 g*
- ➤ *Sugar 2.1 g*
- ➤ *Protein 36.6 g*

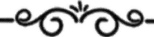

Beef & Black Beans Chili

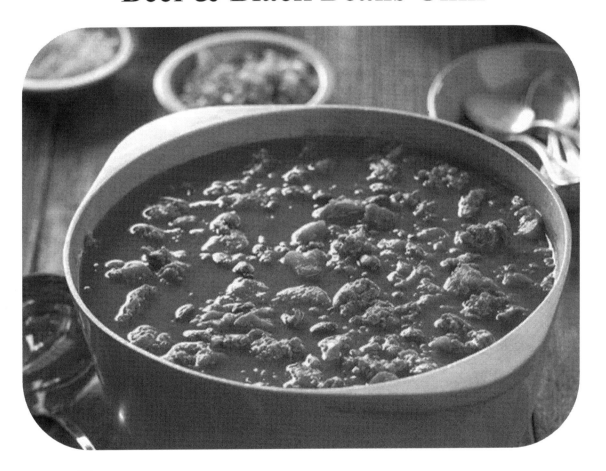

Ingredients

- ➢ 2 pounds lean ground beef
- ➢ 1 tablespoon olive oil
- ➢ 2½ cups green bell pepper, seeded and chopped

- ➤ 1½ cups onion, chopped
- ➤ 2 garlic cloves, minced
- ➤ 1 Serrano pepper, chopped finely
- ➤ ½ tablespoon dried oregano, crushed
- ➤ ½ tablespoon dried thyme, crushed
- ➤ 2 tablespoons red chili powder
- ➤ 1 tablespoon hot paprika
- ➤ 1 tablespoon ground cumin
- ➤ 3 (15-ounce) cans black beans, rinsed and drained
- ➤ 4 cups tomatoes, chopped
- ➤ Water, as needed
- ➤ 8 ounces tomato paste
- ➤ 2 tablespoons balsamic vinegar

How to Prepare

1. Place a Dutch oven over medium heat until heated through.
2. Add beef and cook for about 5–7 minutes or until browned completely.
3. With a slotted spoon, transfer the beef into a bowl.
4. Drain the grease from the pan.
5. In the same pan, heat oil over medium-high heat and sauté the bell pepper and onion for about 5–6 minutes.
6. Add garlic, Serrano pepper, oregano, thyme, and spices, and sauté for about 1 minute.
7. Stir in cooked beef, beans, tomatoes, and enough water to cover and bring to a boil.
8. Stir in tomato paste and again bring to a boil.

9. Now adjust the heat to low and simmer, covered for about 30–35 minutes.

10. Remove the pan of chili from the heat and immediately stir in vinegar.

11. Serve hot.

Preparation time: 15 minutes

Cooking time: 50 minutes

Total time: 1 hour 5 minutes

Servings: 10

Nutritional Values

➤ *Calories 407*

➤ *Total Fat 8.5 g*

➤ *Saturated Fat 2.6 g*

➤ *Cholesterol 81 mg*

➤ *Sodium 105 mg*

➤ *Total Carbs 42.8 g*

➤ *Fiber 14.4 g*

➤ *Sugar 7.1 g*

➤ *Protein 41.3 g*

Beef & Pumpkin Stew

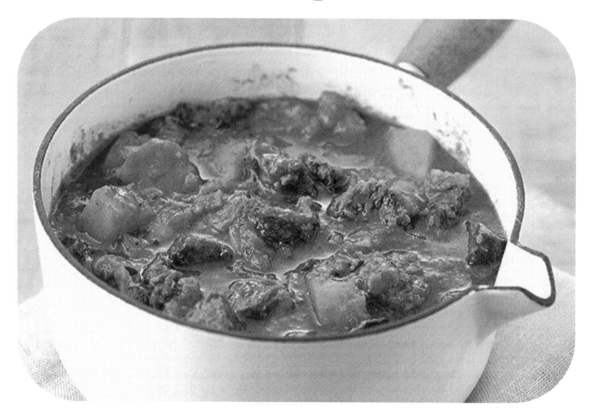

Ingredients

- ➤ 1 pound beef stew meat, trimmed and cubed
- ➤ Salt and ground black pepper, as needed
- ➤ 2 tablespoons extra-virgin olive oil, divided
- ➤ 1 medium carrot, peeled and chopped finely

- ➢ 2 celery stalks, chopped
- ➢ 1 medium onion, chopped
- ➢ 2 cups pumpkin, peeled and cubed
- ➢ 3 cups fresh tomatoes, chopped finely
- ➢ 4 cups water
- ➢ ¼ cup fresh cilantro, chopped

How to Prepare

1. Sprinkle the cubed beef with salt and black pepper evenly.
2. In a large saucepan, heat 1 tablespoon of oil over medium heat and sear beef for about 4–5 minutes.
3. Transfer the beef into a large bowl and set aside.
4. In the same pan, heat the remaining oil over medium heat and sauté carrot, celery, and onion, for about 5 minutes.
5. Add pumpkin and tomatoes and sauté for about 5 minutes.
6. Add water and beef and bring to a boil over high heat.
7. Now adjust the heat to low and simmer, covered for about 1 hour.
8. Uncover and simmer for about 50 minutes.
9. Serve hot with the garnishing of cilantro.

Preparation time: 15 minutes
Cooking time: 2 hours 5 minutes
Total time: 2 hours 20 minutes
Servings: 4

Nutritional Values

➤ Calories 355
➤ Total Fat 14.7 g
➤ Saturated Fat 3.9 g
➤ Cholesterol 101 mg
➤ Sodium 152 mg
➤ Total Carbs 19.5 g
➤ Fiber 6.3 g
➤ Sugar 9.6 g
➤ Protein 37.5 g

SWEET TREAT RECIPES

Chocolaty Cherry Ice Cream

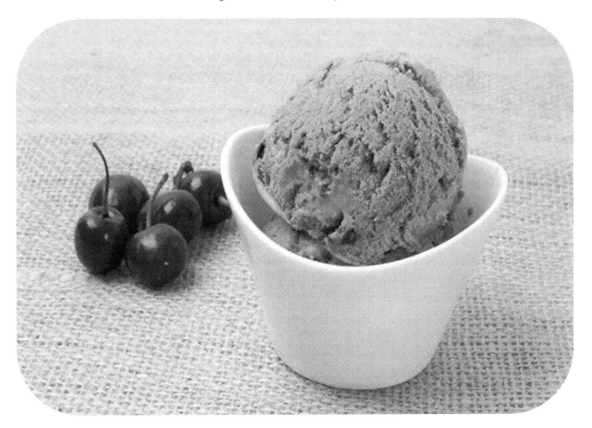

Ingredients
- 1 cup raw cashews
- 1 cup frozen cherries

- ¼ cup unsweetened coconut, shredded
- 1 tablespoon maple syrup
- ¼ cup unsweetened dark chocolate, chopped

How to Prepare

1. In a high-powdered blender, add cashews, and pulse until a flour-like texture forms.
2. Add remaining ingredients (except for chocolate) and pulse until smooth.
3. Add chocolate and pulse until just combined.
4. Transfer the ice-cream into an airtight container and freeze for about 1–2 hours or until set.

Preparation time: 15 minutes
Total time: 15 minutes
Servings: 3

Nutritional Values

- *Calories 460*
- *Total Fat 34.3 g*
- *Saturated Fat 12.9 g*
- *Cholesterol 0 mg*
- *Sodium 16 mg*
- *Total Carbs 31.4 g*
- *Fiber 5.5 g*
- *Sugar 11.3 g*
- *Protein 10.4 g*

Citrus Strawberry Granita

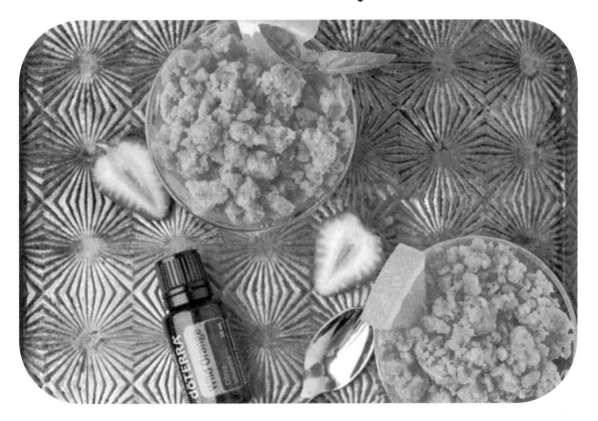

Ingredients
- ➤ 12 ounces fresh strawberries, hulled
- ➤ 1 grapefruit; peeled, seeded, and sectioned
- ➤ 2 oranges; peeled, seeded, and sectioned
- ➤ ¼ of a lemon
- ➤ ¼ cup maple syrup

How to Prepare

1. In a juicer, add strawberries, grapefruit, oranges, and lemon, and process according to manufacturer's directions.

2. In a saucepan, add 1½ cups of the fruit juice and maple syrup over medium heat and cook for about 5 minutes, stirring continuously.

3. Remove the saucepan of juice mixture from heat and stir in the remaining juice.

4. Set aside to cool for about 30 minutes.

5. Transfer the juice mixture into an 8x8-inch glass baking dish.

6. Freeze for about 4 hours, scraping after every 30 minutes.

Preparation time: 15 minutes
Cooking time: 5 minutes
Total time: 20 minutes
Servings: 4

Nutritional Values

➢ *Calories 132*
➢ *Total Fat 0.4 g*
➢ *Saturated Fat 0 g*
➢ *Cholesterol 0 mg*
➢ *Sodium 3 mg*
➢ *Total Carbs 33.2 g*
➢ *Fiber 4.3 g*
➢ *Sugar 26.8 g*
➢ *Protein 1.6 g*

Strawberry Yogurt

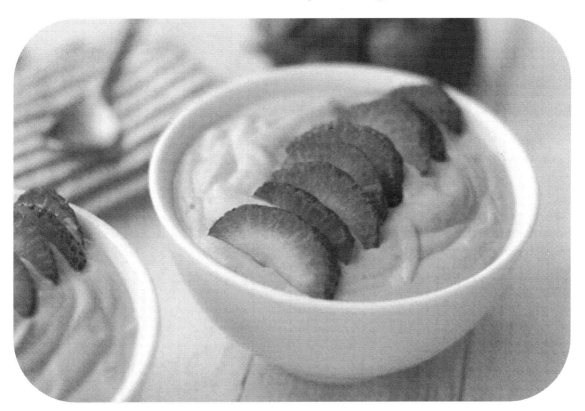

Ingredients

- ➤ 3–5 frozen strawberries
- ➤ 2/3 cup plain fat-free Greek yogurt
- ➤ 1 tablespoon Swerve
- ➤ ½ cup light whipped topping

How to Prepare

1. Place the frozen strawberries in a small microwave-safe bowl and microwave for about 1 minute.

2. Remove from the microwave and with kitchen shears, chop the strawberries finely.

3. Add the yogurt and Swerve and stir to combine.

4. Gently fold in the whipped topping.

5. Serve immediately.

Preparation time: 10 minutes

Cooking time: 1 minute

Total time: 11 minutes

Servings: 4

Nutritional Values

➢ *Calories 53*

➢ *Total Fat 2.2 g*

➢ *Saturated Fat 1.5 g*

➢ *Cholesterol 8 mg*

➢ *Sodium 38 mg*

➢ *Total Carbs 5.1 g*

➢ *Fiber 0.2 g*

➢ *Sugar 4 g*

➢ *Protein 2.5 g*

Chocolate Yogurt Pudding

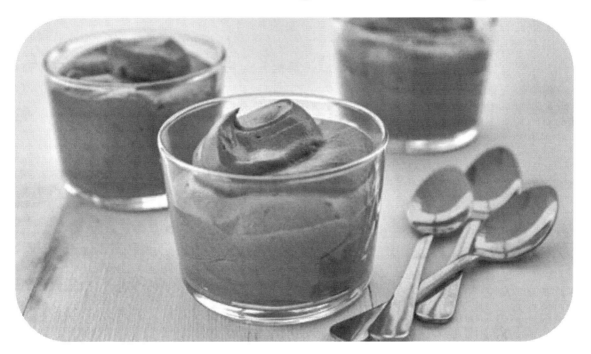

Ingredients

- ➢ 1 cup fat-free plain Greek yogurt
- ➢ 2 tablespoons unsweetened chocolate whey protein powder

How to Prepare

1. In a bowl, put all ingredients and stir to combine.
2. Serve immediately.

Preparation time: 10 minutes

Total time: 10 minutes

Servings: 3

Nutritional Values

- ➢ *Calories 56*
- ➢ *Total Fat 0.4 g*
- ➢ *Saturated Fat 0.2 g*
- ➢ *Cholesterol 9 mg*
- ➢ *Sodium 86 mg*
- ➢ *Total Carbs 6.3 g*
- ➢ *Fiber 0.1 g*
- ➢ *Sugar 0.4 g*
- ➢ *Protein 6.9 g*

Banana Ricotta Pudding

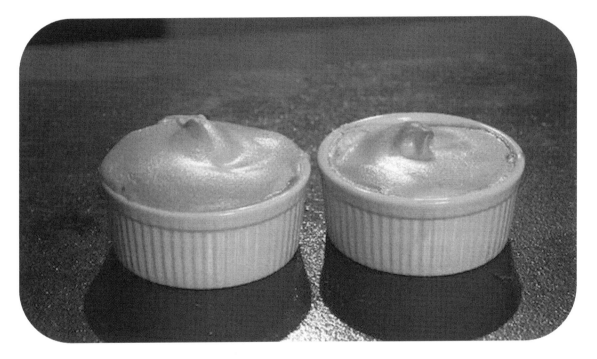

Ingredients

➢ 1 medium ripe banana, peeled

➢ 9 ounces ricotta cheese

➢ 1 egg

How to Prepare

1. Preheat your oven to 375°F.

2. In a bowl, place the banana and mash well.

3. Add the ricotta cheese and egg and mix until well combined.

4. Place the mixture into 3 silicone muffin cups.

5. Bake for approximately 1 hour.

6. Remove the muffin cups from oven and set aside to cool slightly.

7. Serve warm.

Preparation time: 10 minutes
Cooking time: 1 hour
Total time: 1 hour 10 minutes
Servings: 3

Nutritional Values

➢ *Calories 173*
➢ *Total Fat 8.7 g*
➢ *Saturated Fat 4.7 g*
➢ *Cholesterol 81 mg*
➢ *Sodium 127 mg*
➢ *Total Carbs 13.5 g*
➢ *Fiber 1 g*
➢ *Sugar 5.2 g*
➢ *Protein 12 g*

Lemon Pudding

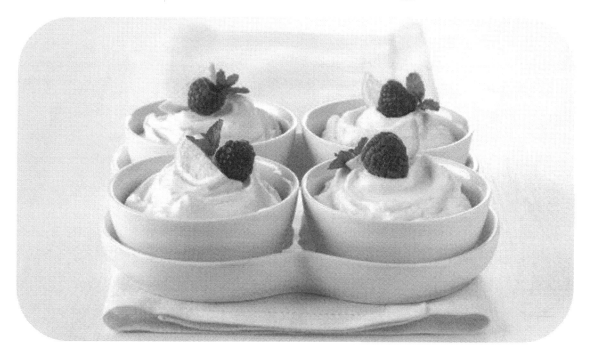

Ingredients

- ➢ 1 small box sugar-free lemon Jell-O
- ➢ ¼ cup hot water
- ➢ ½ cups fat-free plain Greek yogurt
- ➢ 2 scoops unflavored protein powder

How to Prepare

1. In a bowl, place the Jell-O and top with water.
2. Set aside for about 5 minutes.
3. In another bowl, add the yogurt and protein powder and mix well.
4. Transfer the yogurt mixture into the bowl of Jell-O and mix until well combined.
5. Transfer the mixture into ramekins and refrigerate until set before serving.

Preparation time: 10 minutes
Total time: 10 minutes
Servings: 6

Nutritional Values

➢ *Calories 53*
➢ *Total Fat 0.5 g*
➢ *Saturated Fat 0 g*
➢ *Cholesterol 0 mg*
➢ *Sodium 147 mg*
➢ *Total Carbs 1.4 g*
➢ *Fiber 0 g*
➢ *Sugar 0 g*
➢ *Protein 9.9 g*

Chocolate Chia Pudding

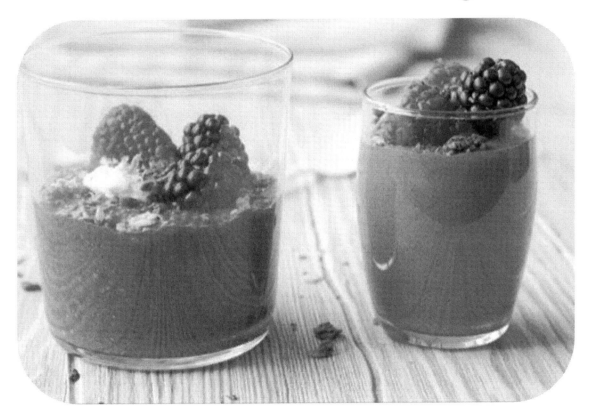

Ingredients

- ➤ 6–9 dates, pitted and chopped
- ➤ 1½ cups unsweetened almond milk
- ➤ 1/3 cup chia seeds
- ➤ ¼ cup cacao powder
- ➤ ½ teaspoon ground cinnamon

> Salt, as needed

> ½ teaspoon vanilla extract

How to Prepare

1. In a food processor, put all ingredients and pulse until smooth.

2. Transfer the mixture into serving bowls.

3. Refrigerate to chill completely before serving.

Preparation time: 10 minutes

Total time: 10 minutes

Servings: 4

Nutritional Values

> *Calories 104*

> *Total Fat 5.7 g*

> *Saturated Fat 1 g*

> *Cholesterol 0 mg*

> *Sodium 107 mg*

> *Total Carbs 16.9 g*

> *Fiber 6.4 g*

> *Sugar 8 g*

> *Protein 3.7 g*

Raspberry Soufflé

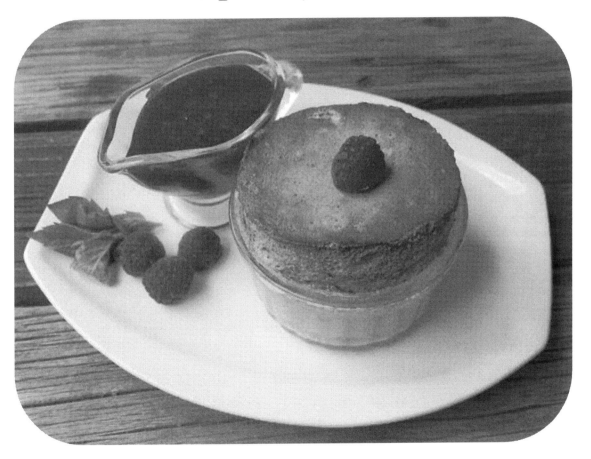

Ingredients
➢ 18 ounces fresh raspberries, hulled

➢ 1/3 cup maple syrup, divided

- ➢ 5 egg whites, divided
- ➢ 4 teaspoons fresh lemon juice

How to Prepare

1. Preheat your oven to 350°F.
2. In a blender, ad raspberries and pulse until a puree forms.
3. Add 3 tablespoons of maple syrup, 2 egg whites, and lemon juice, and pulse until frothy and light.
4. In another bowl, add remaining egg whites and beat until frothy.
5. While beating gradually, add remaining maple syrup and beat until stiff peaks form.
6. Gently, fold the egg whites into the raspberry mixture.
7. Transfer the mixture into 6 large ramekins evenly.
8. Arrange the ramekins into a baking sheet.
9. Bake for approximately 10–12 minutes.
10. Serve immediately.

Preparation time: 15 minutes
Cooking time: 12 minutes
Total time: 27 minutes
Servings: 6

Nutritional Values

- ➢ *Calories 105*
- ➢ *Total Fat 0.7 g*
- ➢ *Saturated Fat 0.1 g*

- ➤ *Cholesterol 0 mg*
- ➤ *Sodium 31 mg*
- ➤ *Total Carbs 22.2 g*
- ➤ *Fiber 5.5 g*
- ➤ *Sugar 14.4 g*
- ➤ *Protein 4.1 g*

Chocolate Lava Cake

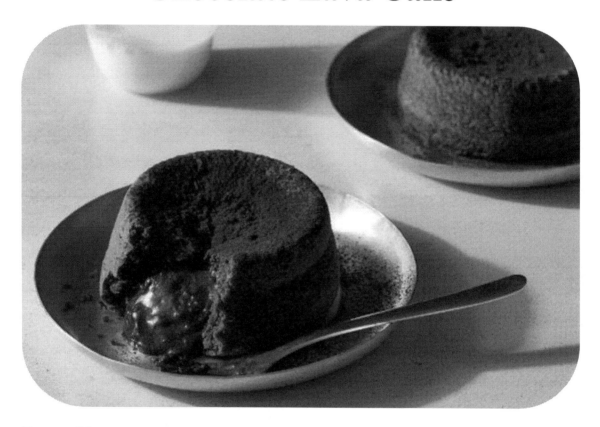

Ingredients

- ➤ 3 tablespoons coconut oil
- ➤ 4 ounce unsweetened dark chocolate, chopped
- ➤ 2 tablespoons maple syrup
- ➤ 2 eggs

- ➢ ½ teaspoon vanilla extract
- ➢ Pinch of salt
- ➢ 1 tablespoon cacao powder
- ➢ 1 tablespoon almond flour

How to Prepare

1. Preheat your oven to 375°F.
2. Grease 4 ramekins and dust with a little cocoa powder. Arrange ramekins in a large baking sheet.
3. In a large microwave-safe bowl, mix together coconut oil and chocolate.
4. Microwave on high for about 1–1½ minutes or until melted and combined completely, stirring occasionally.
5. In another bowl, add maple syrup, eggs, vanilla, and salt, and beat until well combined.
6. Add the coconut oil mixture and stir until well combined.
7. Add almond flour and cocoa powder and mix until well combined.
8. Transfer the mixture into prepared ramekins evenly.
9. Bake for approximately 10–12 minutes.
10. Remove the ramekins from oven and set aside for about 1–2 minutes.
11. Carefully invert the cakes onto the serving plates serve.

Preparation time: 10 minutes
Cooking time: 13½ minutes
Total time: 23½ minutes
Servings: 4

Nutritional Values

- ➢ Calories 350
- ➢ Total Fat 28.7 g
- ➢ Saturated Fat 19.2 g
- ➢ Cholesterol 82 mg
- ➢ Sodium 80 mg
- ➢ Total Carbs 15.5 g
- ➢ Fiber 4.4 g
- ➢ Sugar 6.3 g
- ➢ Protein 6.8 g

Grilled Peaches

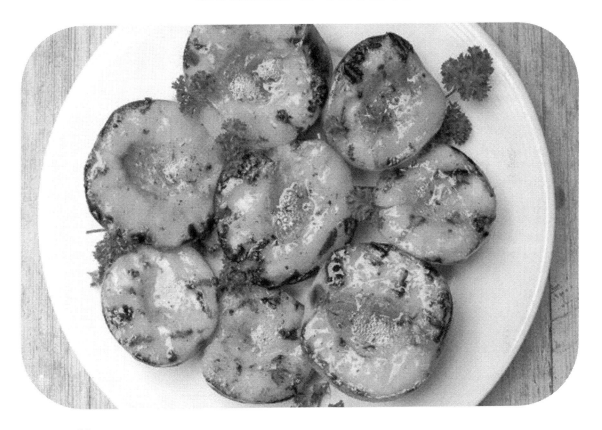

Ingredients
- ➤ 3 medium peaches, halved and pitted
- ➤ Ground cinnamon, as needed

How to Prepare

1. Preheat the grill to medium-low heat.

2. Grease the grill grate.

3. Arrange the peach slices onto the grill, cut-side down.

4. Grill for about 3–5 minutes per side or until desired doneness.

5. Sprinkle with cinnamon and serve.

Preparation time: 10 minutes

Total time: 10 minutes

Servings: 6

Nutritional Values

- ➤ *Calories 30*
- ➤ *Total Fat 0.2 g*
- ➤ *Saturated Fat 0 g*
- ➤ *Cholesterol 0 mg*
- ➤ *Sodium 0 mg*
- ➤ *Total Carbs 7 g*
- ➤ *Fiber 1.2 g*
- ➤ *Sugar 7 g*
- ➤ *Protein 0.7 g*

DRESSING, SAUCES & SEASONING RECIPES

Greek Dressing

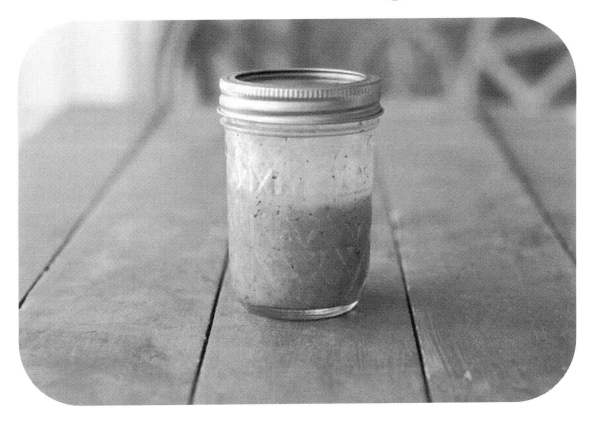

Ingredients
➤ 1 garlic clove, minced

- ¼ cup extra-virgin olive oil
- 2 tablespoons fresh lemon juice
- 1 teaspoon dried oregano, crushed
- ¼ teaspoon salt
- ¼ teaspoon freshly ground black pepper

How to Prepare

1. In a bowl, add all ingredients and beat until well combined.
2. Transfer the dressing into an airtight jar and store in the refrigerator.

Preparation time: 10 minutes
Total time: 10 minutes
Servings: 4

Nutritional Values

- *Calories 112*
- *Total Fat 12.7 g*
- *Saturated Fat 1.9 g*
- *Cholesterol 0 mg*
- *Sodium 149 mg*
- *Total Carbs 0.7 g*
- *Fiber 0.2 g*
- *Sugar 0.2 g*
- *Protein 0.2 g*

Strawberry Dressing

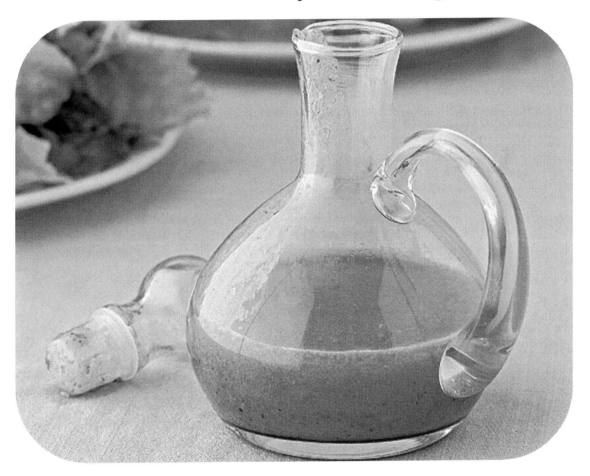

Ingredients
- ➤ ½ cup fresh strawberries, hulled and sliced
- ➤ ½ cup olive oil

- ➤ 2 tablespoons balsamic vinegar
- ➤ 1 teaspoon pure maple syrup
- ➤ 1 teaspoon mustard
- ➤ 1 teaspoon salt
- ➤ 1 teaspoon freshly ground black pepper

How to Prepare

1. In a high-powered blender, add strawberries and pulse until pureed.
2. Now add remaining ingredients and pulse until smooth and creamy.
3. Transfer the dressing into an airtight jar and store in the refrigerator.

Preparation time: 10 minutes
Total time: 10 minutes
Servings: 8

Nutritional Values

- ➤ *Calories 116*
- ➤ *Total Fat 12.8 g*
- ➤ *Saturated Fat 1.8 g*
- ➤ *Cholesterol 0 mg*
- ➤ *Sodium 291 mg*
- ➤ *Total Carbs 1.6 g*
- ➤ *Fiber 0.3 g*
- ➤ *Sugar 1 g*
- ➤ *Protein 2.1 g*

Tomato Dressing

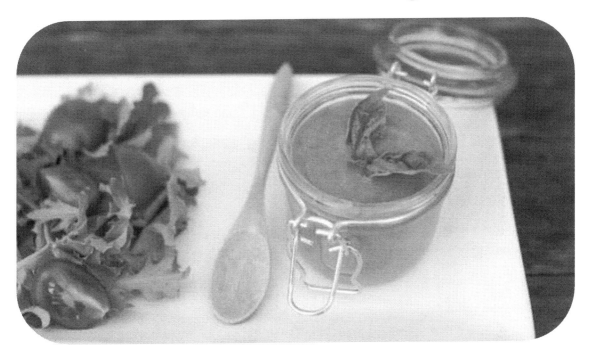

Ingredients

- ➤ 1 large tomato, chopped roughly
- ➤ 2 garlic cloves, chopped
- ➤ ½ cup olive oil
- ➤ 2 tablespoons fresh lemon juice
- ➤ 1 packet stevia
- ➤ 1 tablespoon dried thyme, crushed
- ➤ 1 tablespoon dried tarragon, crushed

- ➤ ½ teaspoon paprika
- ➤ Salt, as needed

How to Prepare

1. In a high-powered blender, put all ingredients and pulse until smooth.

2. Serve immediately.

Preparation time: 10 minutes

Total time: 10 minutes

Servings: 4

Nutritional Values

- ➤ *Calories 232*
- ➤ *Total Fat 25.5 g*
- ➤ *Saturated Fat 3.7 g*
- ➤ *Cholesterol 0 mg*
- ➤ *Sodium 44 mg*
- ➤ *Total Carbs 3.1 g*
- ➤ *Fiber 1 g*
- ➤ *Sugar 1.4 g*
- ➤ *Protein 0.8 g*

Avocado Dressing

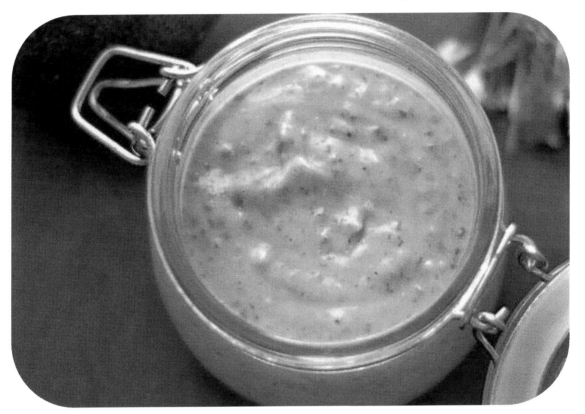

Ingredients

- ¾ cup fresh cilantro, chopped
- ½ of medium avocado, peeled, pitted and chopped
- 2 medium onions, chopped
- 1 garlic clove, chopped

- ¼ cup unsweetened coconut milk
- 1/3 cup avocado oil
- 2 tablespoons fresh lime juice
- ½ teaspoon salt
- ½ teaspoon freshly ground black pepper

How to Prepare

1. In a high-powered blender, put all ingredients and pulse until smooth.

2. Transfer the dressing into an airtight jar and store in the refrigerator.

Preparation time: 10 minutes

Total time: 10 minutes

Servings: 8

Nutritional Values

- *Calories 136*
- *Total Fat 13.4 g*
- *Saturated Fat 3.2 g*
- *Cholesterol 0 mg*
- *Sodium 151 mg*
- *Total Carbs 4.4 g*
- *Fiber 1.7 g*
- *Sugar 1.5 g*
- *Protein 0.8 g*

Cherry & Cranberry Sauce

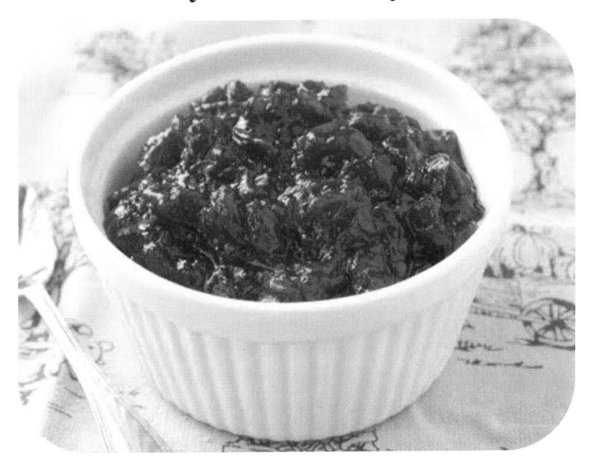

Ingredients
- ➤ 6 ounces frozen cherries
- ➤ 6 ounces frozen cranberries
- ➤ ½ teaspoon fresh ginger, minced

- ¾ cup fresh apple juice
- Pinch of salt
- ¼ teaspoon ground cinnamon
- 1-2 tablespoons maple syrup

How to Prepare

1. In a saucepan, mix together cherries, cranberries, ginger, apple juice, and salt over high heat and bring to a boil.
2. Now adjust the heat to medium and simmer for about 8–10 minutes, stirring occasionally.
3. Stir in cinnamon and maple syrup and remove from heat.

Preparation time: 10 minutes
Cooking time: 10 minutes
Total time: 20 minutes
Servings: 8

Nutritional Values
- *Calories 54*
- *Total Fat 0.1 g*
- *Saturated Fat 0 g*
- *Cholesterol 0 mg*
- *Sodium 24 mg*
- *Total Carbs 12.3 g*
- *Fiber 1 g*
- *Sugar 4.5 g*
- *Protein 0.1 g*

BBQ Sauce

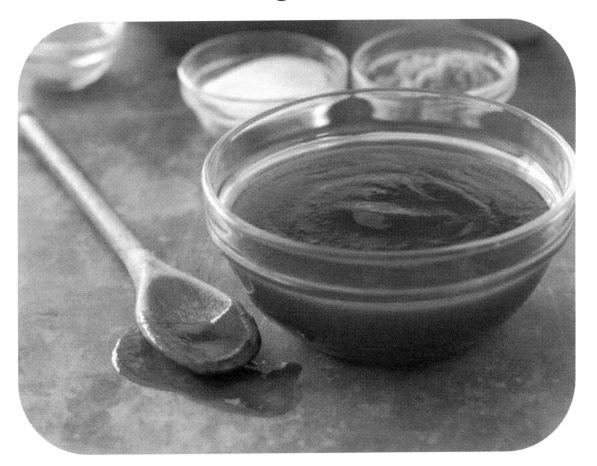

Ingredients

➢ 16 ounces tomato sauce

➢ ½ cup apple cider vinegar

➢ 5 tablespoons maple syrup

- ➢ 2 tablespoons tomato paste
- ➢ 1 tablespoon fresh lemon juice
- ➢ ½ tablespoon ground mustard
- ➢ ½ tablespoon onion powder
- ➢ ½ tablespoons ground black pepper
- ➢ 1 teaspoon paprika
- ➢ 1 cup water

How to Prepare

1. In a saucepan, mix together all ingredients over medium-high heat and bring to a gentle boil.
2. Now adjust the heat to low and simmer for about 1 hour or until desired thickness.
3. Remove the saucepan of sauce from heat and transfer into an airtight container.
4. Set aside to cool completely before storing in the refrigerator.

Preparation time: 15 minutes
Cooking time: 1 hour 5 minutes
Total time: 1 hour 20 minutes
Servings: 12

Nutritional Values

- ➢ *Calories 40*
- ➢ *Total Fat 0.3 g*
- ➢ *Saturated Fat 0 g*

- ➢ *Cholesterol 0 mg*
- ➢ *Sodium 203 mg*
- ➢ *Total Carbs 8.9 g*
- ➢ *Fiber 0.9 g*
- ➢ *Sugar 7.1 g*
- ➢ *Protein 0.8 g*

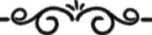

Mustard Sauce

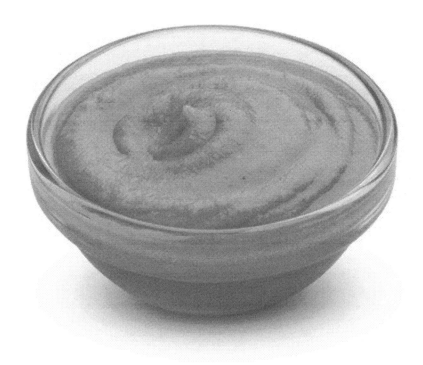

Ingredients

> ½ cup stone-ground mustard

> ¼ cup balsamic vinegar

> ¼ cup maple syrup

How to Prepare

1. In a bowl, add all ingredients and beat until well combined.

2. Refrigerate before serving.

Preparation time: 10 minutes
Total time: 10 minutes
Servings: 16

Nutritional Values

➢ *Calories 37*
➢ *Total Fat 1.4 g*
➢ *Saturated Fat 0.1 g*
➢ *Cholesterol 0 mg*
➢ *Sodium 1 mg*
➢ *Total Carbs 5.1 g*
➢ *Fiber 0.7 g*
➢ *Sugar 3.3 g*
➢ *Protein 1.2 g*

Almond Butter

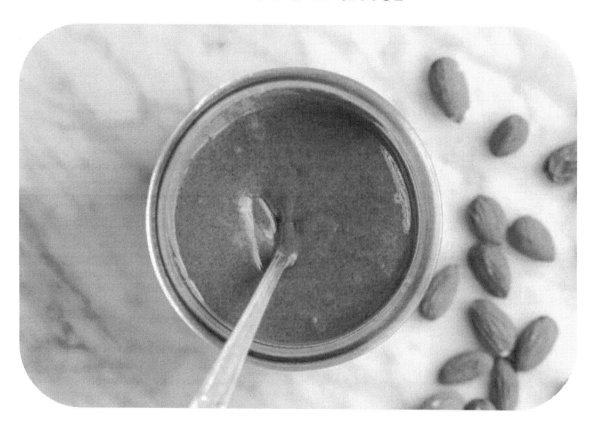

Ingredients

➤ 2¼ cups raw almonds

➤ 1 tablespoon coconut oil

➤ ¾ teaspoon salt

➤ 2 tablespoons maple syrup

➤ ½ teaspoon ground cinnamon

How to Prepare

1. Preheat your oven to 325°F.
2. Arrange the almonds onto a rimmed baking sheet.
3. Bake for approximately 12–15 minutes.
4. Remove from oven and set aside to cool completely.
5. In a food processor, fitted with a metal blade, add almonds and pulse until a fine meal forms.
6. Add coconut oil and salt and pulse for about 6–9 minutes.
7. Add maple syrup and cinnamon and pulse for about 1–2 minutes.
8. Transfer the almond butter in an airtight jar and store in refrigerator.

Preparation time: 15 minutes
Cooking time: 15 minutes
Total time: 30 minutes
Servings: 6

Nutritional Values

➤ *Calories 244*
➤ *Total Fat 20.1 g*
➤ *Saturated Fat 3.3 g*
➤ *Cholesterol 0 mg*
➤ *Sodium 292 mg*
➤ *Total Carbs 12.3 g*
➤ *Fiber 4.6 g*
➤ *Sugar 5.5 g*
➤ *Protein 7.6 g*

Green Curry Paste

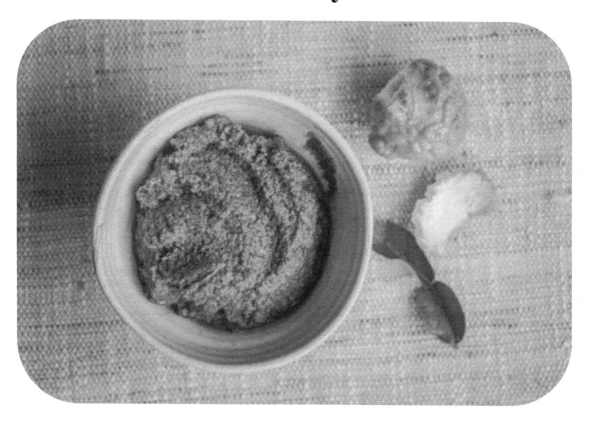

Ingredients
- ➤ 2 shallots, chopped roughly
- ➤ 1 tablespoon fresh ginger, chopped roughly
- ➤ 4 garlic cloves, chopped roughly
- ➤ 1 fresh lemongrass stalk

- ➢ 2 teaspoons fresh lime zest
- ➢ 3–6 Serrano peppers, seeded and chopped
- ➢ ¾ cup fresh cilantro, chopped roughly
- ➢ ½ cup fresh basil leaves, chopped
- ➢ 1 teaspoon ground coriander
- ➢ 1 teaspoon ground cumin
- ➢ 2 teaspoons paprika
- ➢ 1 teaspoon salt
- ➢ 1 tablespoon fresh lime juice
- ➢ 1 tablespoon coconut aminos

How to Prepare

1. In a high-powered food processor, add all ingredients and pulse until smooth paste forms.
2. Preserve in an airtight container.

Preparation time: 10 minutes
Total time: 10 minutes
Servings: 8

Nutritional Values

- ➢ *Calories 14*
- ➢ *Total Fat 0.2 g*
- ➢ *Saturated Fat 0 g*
- ➢ *Cholesterol 0mg*
- ➢ *Sodium 296 mg*
- ➢ *Total Carbs 3 g*

- Fiber 0.5 g
- Sugar 0.2 g
- Protein 0.6 g

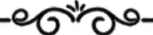

Taco Seasoning

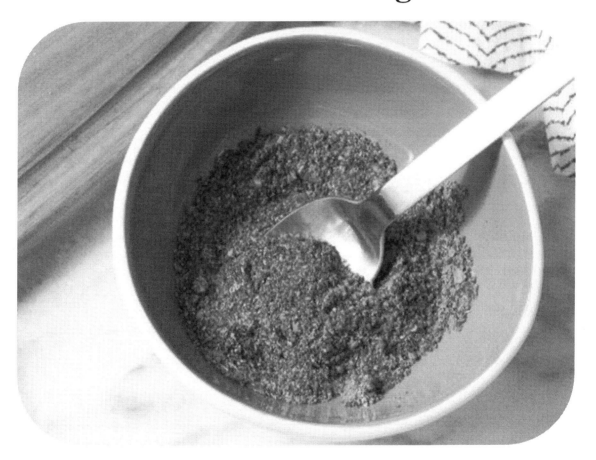

Ingredients
- ➤ 1 tablespoon red chili powder
- ➤ 1½ teaspoons ground cumin
- ➤ ½ teaspoon paprika
- ➤ ¼ teaspoon dried oregano, crushed

- ¼ teaspoon red pepper flakes, crushed
- ¼ teaspoon garlic powder
- ¼ teaspoon onion powder
- Salt and ground black pepper, as needed

How to Prepare

1. In a bowl, mix together all ingredients.

2. Store in an airtight jar.

Preparation time: 5 minutes

Total time: 5 minutes

Servings: 10

Nutritional Values

- *Calories 5*
- *Total Fat 0.2 g*
- *Saturated Fat 0 g*
- *Cholesterol 0 mg*
- *Sodium 24 mg*
- *Total Carbs 0.8 g*
- *Fiber 0.4 g*
- *Sugar 0.1 g*
- *Protein 0.2 g*

CHAPTER 4: CONVERSION TABLES

Oven Temperature

Fahrenheit	Centigrade
250	120
300	150
325	160
350	180
375	180
400	190
450	200
500	250

Mass

Imperial (ounces)	Metric (gram)
¼ ounce	7 grams
½ ounce	14 grams
1 ounce	28 grams
2 ounces	56 grams
3 ounces	85 grams

4 ounces	113 grams
5 ounces	141 grams
6 ounces	150 grams
7 ounces	198 grams
8 ounces	226 grams
9 ounces	255 grams
10 ounces	283 grams
11 ounces	311 grams
12 ounces	340 grams
13 ounces	368 grams
14 ounces	396 grams
15 ounces	425 grams
16 ounces/ 1 pound	455 grams

Cups & Spoons

Cups	Metric
¼ cup	60 milliliters
1/3 cup	80 milliliters
½ cup	120 milliliters
1 cup	240 milliliters
Spoon	**Metric**
¼ teaspoon	1¼ milliliters
½ teaspoon	2½ milliliters
1 teaspoon	5 milliliters
2 teaspoons	10 milliliters
1 tablespoon	20 milliliters

Liquid

Imperial	Metric
1 fluid ounce	30 milliliters
2 fluid ounces	60 milliliters
3½ fluid ounces	80 milliliters
2¾ fluid ounces	100 milliliters
4 fluid ounces	125 milliliters
5 fluid ounces	150 milliliters
6 fluid ounces	180 milliliters
7 fluid ounces	200 milliliters
8¾ fluid ounces	250 milliliters
10½ fluid ounces	310 milliliters
13 fluid ounces	375 milliliters
15 fluid ounces	430 milliliters
16 fluid ounces	475 milliliters
17 fluid ounces	500 milliliters
21½ fluid ounces	625 milliliters
26 fluid ounces	750 milliliters
35 fluid ounces	1 Liter
44 fluid ounces	1¼ Liters
52 fluid ounces	1½ Liters
70 fluid ounces	2 Liters
88 fluid ounces	2½ Liters

CONCLUSION

Perhaps, weight loss can be achieved when we provide the body with just enough calories to meet the nutritional needs and nothing more than that. The caloric restriction can be maintained by controlling the dietary patterns or reducing the amount of food intake. Some people simply cannot afford to make the dietary changes, so they can take benefit from gastric sleeve surgery to reduce daily food consumption and achieve weight loss in no time. Sleeve gastrectomy, or the gastric sleeve treatment, is a restrictive operation that can limit the stomach size and reduce its food holding capacity. Do that; the patient would feel fuller and eat less food at a time. Usually, a person has the size of a stomach according to their body size, and it is needed. It is large enough to hold food for a longer duration to prevent any food deficiency emergency. This procedure includes the removal of about 2/3 of the stomach. Don't worry! The stomach is not literally removed; rather, this portion is only separated or parted from the other 1/3 portion. The surgeon staples or sews the walls of the stomach to divide it into these two parts. The 1/3 part connects the cardiac sphincter with the pyloric sphincter; thus, the food comes in and soon leaves the stomach after partial digestion. After this surgery, only a vertical tube of the stomach, almost about the size of a banana, is left functional. Changing the natural stomach size can only prove healthy if this surgery is considered a tool to achieve weight and not a quick fix for all your health problems. Gastric sleeve surgery changes a person's life altogether. Therefore, it requires a special diet to support the changes. In this cook, we have shared all the suitable bariatric diet recipes to make it easier for those going through post-op complications.

Made in United States
Orlando, FL
10 December 2021

11437427R00176